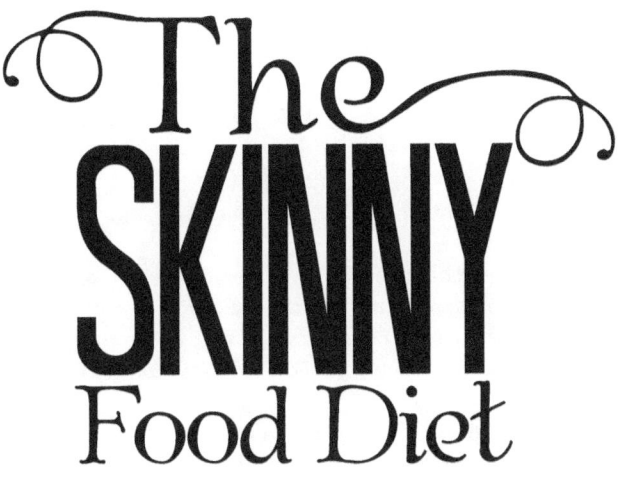

The
SKINNY
Food Diet

A DELICIOUS PARODY

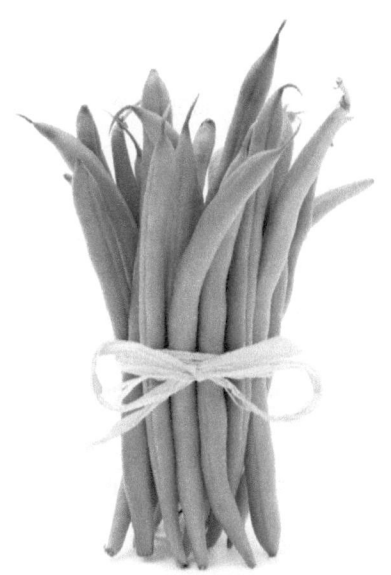

Caduceus Twigg, PhT

ISBN: 978-1-4834-8844-8 (sc)
ISBN: 978-1-4834-8843-1 (e)

Library of Congress Control Number: 2018908304

Lulu Publishing Services rev. date: 9/18/2018

Contents

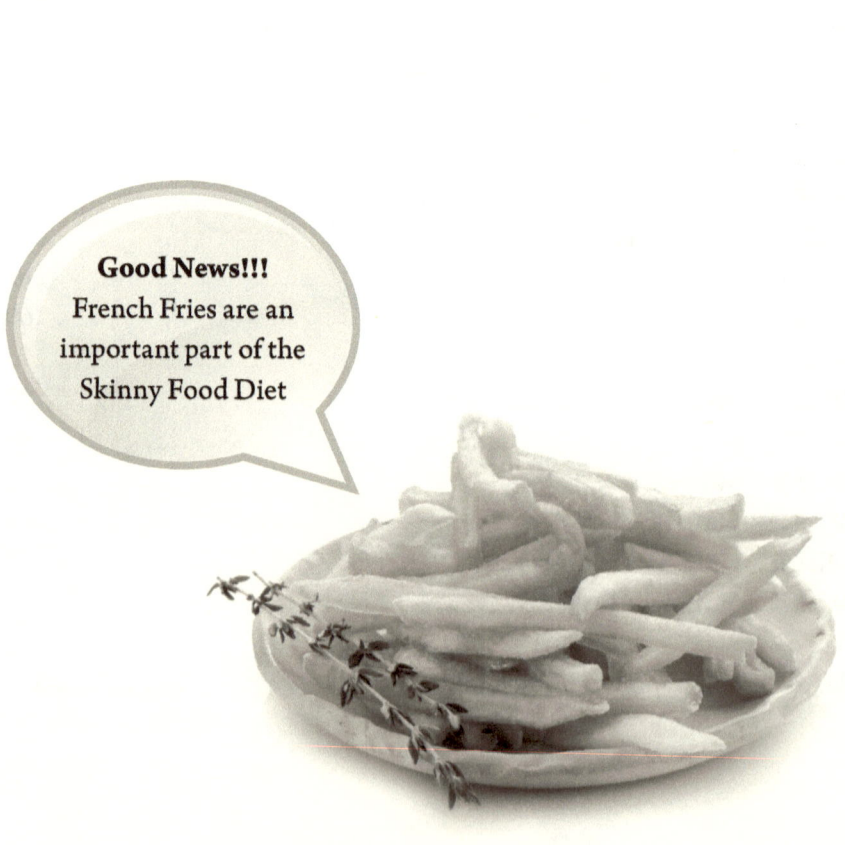

Good News!!!
French Fries are an important part of the Skinny Food Diet

Preface

In the beginning, there was Lunch, and Lunch was good. However, Lunch was lonely and wanted a friend, for as we all know, it is no fun to eat by yourself. And since Lunch was all alone, Breakfast was created. Lunch loved Breakfast. She had a sweet sunny-side-up disposition. With her, it was always orange juice and champagne, caviar and cream cheese. Lunch couldn't keep his eyes off her. And since they lay together on the same table, it wasn't too long before their child, Brunch, was born.

Breakfast loved Brunch and Brunch loved Breakfast. It was as though they were made to be on the menu together. However, as time went on Brunch become more and more like his father - bigger, heavier, and even a little overweight. Pretty soon Breakfast could no longer recognize her small, sweet son. Breakfast and Lunch fought. "Brunch will never come between us," said Lunch, trying desperately to hold on to Breakfast. But in the end, Breakfast and Lunch separated. Brunch would have weekend visitation.

Breakfast was sad but soon found comfort on the late night menu. It is here that she met Dinner. Suave and debonair, Dinner had all the right moves. He knew wine and cognac, cigars and cappuccinos. Here, she found everything that Lunch wasn't. Sure, Lunch was reasonably priced, but where was the excitement, the passion, the joy? Soon Breakfast and Dinner were spending every night together and it wasn't long before they, too, consummated their love and Midnight was born.

Breakfast and Dinner were "over the moon" with the arrival of Midnight. They loved her desperately, and doted on her as new parents often do. They were a happy family. The years passed and one day Midnight told her parents that it was time for her to leave their table. She loved them dearly, but she needed to see the world, to experience new things, and get a job. Casting about for interesting opportunities, she found just what she was looking for on a cruise ship. When she was introduced to the captain he said, "I know your parents Breakfast and Dinner, but I don't believe we've had the pleasure." To which she replied, "My name is Midnight, Midnight Buffet".

And that is the story of how Breakfast, Brunch, Lunch, Dinner, and Midnight Buffet came to be the one big family that we all love. In fact, we love them so much that we take them with us wherever we go. We add them to our waistlines, hips, thighs, and bellies. They make our shoes tighter, our airplane seats smaller and our closets fuller. Try as we might we can't live without them. It is time to face facts - we are in love with food.

What is the modern man and woman to do with our love for food? We can skip meals, go on cleansing regimens, try any one of a 100 diets or work-out until we drop. Yet, you and I both know that none of these approaches will give us the shape we are seeking. Most adults in the western world are overweight and in many cases obese. If it was easy to say "not tonight" to Dinner, we would be thin already. No, the answer to becoming thin is to take an entirely new approach to eating, one based on an overlooked area of food science and nutrition, one that is easy to understand, easy to follow, and delicious. In fact, you can explain it to a 6-year-old and they "get it." What is this miracle you ask? It is a diet based on food shape. Yes, food shape.

Scientists and researchers, the world over will wonder why they hadn't thought of this sooner. By focusing on carbohydrates, fats, sugars, time of day, or food they missed the obvious connection between food shape and your shape. What could be simpler? However, before we are too hard on these folks, maybe, these PhDs and MDs have done humanity a great favor by showing us what doesn't work? Throw out all your other diet books, there is a new diet in town and it's called "The Skinny Food Diet."

"Skinny foods for breakfast?" Bring it on! "Skinny foods for lunch?" No problem! How about Skinny Foods for dinner, brunch, and midnight buffet? Love it! Eat all you want. No matter what meal you choose, we have got Skinny Foods for you. And, by eating Skinny Foods for 3-4 meals per day you will lose those extra pounds, becoming the thin "you" that you know you are. And once you lose the weight, maintenance is simple - just eat Skinny Foods for 1-2 meals per day and you will keep your beautiful new shape. Whether it is breakfast, lunch, brunch, dinner or midnight buffet, you just eat your way to becoming thin. What could be easier?

~ Caduceus

Chapter 1

WHY THIN IS ALWAYS "IN"

Hey "Toothpick", "String Bean" or "Skeleton," how many times did you hear that as a child? For me, it was a lot, and it felt pretty good. Of course these days, no one, except politicians, get away with public name-calling, but when we were young, the playground was open season on those of us who were a little bit different. However, as adults, we seldom hear those words. We're more likely to hear under-the-breath comments like "piggy," "porky" and "lard-ass," and these comments really do hurt. It seems that we just can't win. One minute we are thin and gorgeous, and the next we are fat. What is going on?

Let's go back to the playground when most of us were thin. We were thin because we were using the energy from our food to perform all the physical activities of youth. Whether it was learning new things such as walking, speaking, running, reading, texting or just growing, we were burning up most all of the calories we consumed. But what happens when we quit running, slow our learning, and stop growing? When we find the couch more fun than the swing or a basketball game is only something to watch on TV. It is then we find that foods we consume can turn into those few extra pounds, which over a lifetime turn into a huge weight problem.

"Work out more" is the popular mantra of the health and diet industry. As if a few trips to the gym could be enough to solve the world's obesity problem. Unfortunately, exercise is not the answer. To illustrate this point, let me share a personal story. A number of years ago, I was approached by a friend to help with a local triathlon event, "The Vineman," in Sonoma County, California. This race offers the full triathlon, a half triathlon, and a run for breast cancer. I agreed to help out as long as I could have a "good" job. I wasn't too interested in the typical volunteer jobs such as parking cars or moving equipment. And to this, my friend said, "I have the perfect job for a man of your talents." With a compliment like that, who could resist? What was the amazing job you might ask? It was helping contestants remove their wetsuits after the swimming portion of the triathlon. Sound like fun? It was. By the way, in case you are wondering, some folks really do go "commando" (naked) under their wetsuits.

The reason that I bring up this story is that the athletes competing in the Vineman came in all body types. Lots of folks were thin and svelte, but there were many who were a bit overweight for their height. Now, to compete in a triathlon, these athletes had been training for many months. Some were working out three hours a day, six days a week. Starting with a daily, half-mile swim, most would then go on to an afternoon bike ride or run. Just their running schedule alone would be enough to give most folks heart palpitations, something like 50 miles per week towards the end of their training period. In other words, here were athletes at the peak of their physical performance and some were still overweight. Clearly, working out isn't enough when it comes to weight loss. You can be in great muscular and cardiovascular shape but still be overweight.

Even if you are exercising every day, you may still have trouble keeping those extra pounds off. This has much to do with living in the super-abundant 21st century. It was Wallis Simpson, the wife of King Edward of England, who was purported to say, "You can never be too rich or too thin." She was clearly on to something here. In ancient times, it was a sign of wealth to be heavy. When food was scarce, it was only the wealthy who had enough to eat. They were the ones who could afford calorie-rich foods such as meat, fruits, butter, cheese and other fats. They were the ones who didn't have to work very hard and could enjoy their leisure. Conversely, poorer folks had to work hard for the little money they earned, and then could only afford a few calories in the form of flour, grains, or potatoes. Fresh meat for the poor was a rare thing and greatly treasured. So, the rich were fat and the poor were thin.

As Mrs. Simpson noted in the 20th century, this all changed, now it is the rich who are thin and the poor who are fat. How did this happen? It is a complex situation. However, there are a couple of things that are fairly obvious. First, in the markets of today, fruits and vegetables generally cost much more than processed foods. And, if you have a limited budget, and need to feed yourself and/or your family, you are likely to buy the calorie-rich foods (sweetened cereals, donuts, muffins, and cookies) that cost less. These foods will fill you up, but often lack the fiber and nutrients for a healthy diet.

Additionally, if you are of more limited means, you might be tempted to access government-commodity food programs. Here, you will find "gov'ment cheese" and other high-calorie commodities such as peanut butter. While there are plenty of healthy choices in these government programs, we are all drawn to fat, sugar, and salt and who can resist free cheese?

Then there is the whole subject of fast food. Even now the fast food chains are experimenting with drone delivery. Someday, you won't need to get off your couch for the pizza delivery. Just leave a window open, and a drone-delivered dinner will come right to your recliner.

Much has been written about the many health benefits of being thin. By keeping your weight under control you can avoid many of the plagues of modernity such as high blood pressure, heart disease, diabetes, and cancer to name a few. It seems like every few weeks another report is issued by a government lab decrying the problems with our favorite foods. Processed meats, barbecued meats, sodium, triglycerides, tropical oils, the list goes on and on. Sometimes it is hard for the average consumer to know what is good and what is bad. What we do know is that carrying those extra pounds in not healthy. If nothing else, just the stress on your joints may be enough to remind you that your knees and hips weren't designed for hauling heavy loads.

If you couldn't remember this on your own, the popular media is there to remind you that "thin is in." In fact, for the past 100 years or so, thin has never been "out." Recall Popeye and Olive Oyl from the 1930's. Olive is the 'poster child" for thin. Having perfectly proportioned measurements of 17, 17, 17, she was the love interest of Popeye and as good and wholesome a girl as you could imagine. Brutus, on the other hand, was fat, slovenly and the enemy of all goodness. And as Popeye continually bested Brutus to claim the hand Olive, the moral imperative of "thin" winning over "fat" was clear to all.

Even as tastes changed, "thin" is still the thing to be. It is a little-known fact that the hippy movement of the 1960's was not about the need to fight repression at home or the U.S. involvement in Vietnam abroad. Nor was it a counter-culture revolution, led by high-minded idealists looking for some utopian existence. No, it was all about men and women coming together to lose the pounds that had accumulated since the Great Depression. The post-war WWII era was one of abundance of food, and for the first time in history the dining table was filled. Twiggy, and her thin contemporaries, were the counter argument to this time of abundance, suggesting that you didn't have to eat all the food that was put in front of you.

Of course, American food companies are pros at getting their customers hooked on unhealthy foods. As soon as children turn on the TV, they are inundated with commercials from the cereal and snack food companies. American children see as many as 10,000 commercials in their young lives and many of these commercials are promoting sweetened cereals, chips, candy, and sodas. But we can fight back. Even children understand that not all foods are healthy. Just look at Sesame Street, Kermit and simple-minded Ernie showed us how to take on the Cookie Monster and Miss Piggy and win. Miss Piggy can't ever get Kermit to the altar, and Cookie Monsters gluttony can never be satisfied. Good triumphs over evil and in the case of the Muppets, thin wins over fat.

And, deep down, we all want to be thin. We want to fight the forces of modernity that shove calorie after calorie into our world. We must tell the food producers that being 50 lbs. overweight is not our natural state. Humans evolved to be tall and thin, to run for days chasing down prey animals and to live in warm climates without the need to accumulate an extra layer of fat. No, the answer to those extra pounds that we all carry around is to return to our beginnings, starting with our diet.

What is a healthful diet? It one that supports our caloric needs while reinforcing the image of the body type that we are seeking.

If you want to be thin, then logic and science dictate that you should consume thin foods. That means a diet thin on calories, thin on fats, thin on sugars and thin on you. It is the Skinny Food Diet.

Like many other important discoveries, the Skinny Food Diet was hiding in plain sight. Skinny foods such as carrots, bananas, celery, and the all-important, skinny, super foods like asparagus, have been around for centuries. However, it wasn't until I observed the powerful and synergistic connection between these foods that the Skinny Food Diet was born.

Sometimes all it takes is looking at a problem or situation in a new way and the answer becomes obvious.

For example, Newton may have been a brilliant man, but he didn't invent gravity. Gravity existed since time began, however Newton was the first to explain it mathematically after watching an apple fall to the ground. Similarly, Darwin, on his voyage to the Pacific, noticed the variations in finches on the Galapagos Islands and expounded the Theory of Evolution. So, too, the Skinny Food Diet has been discovered by a careful examination of the qualities and healthfulness of skinny foods. And, like the theories of gravity and evolution, the Theory of Thin has a significant scientific basis that serves to explain the phenomena, and provides scientists and researchers, working in the field, the ability to create new, super skinny foods.

The following pages will make the case for the Skinny Food Diet. First, I will construct a new paradigm for the outdated metric of the Body Mass Index (BMI). The proposed metric, the Body Height Index or (BHI) is a superior way to answer the age-old question of "What is my ideal height?" I will then show a rigorous scientific model using formulas and advanced math to determine the goodness of foods or the Food Health Index (FHI), based on their physical dimensions. (Readers will be shocked to learn that some of our most cherished foods, apples for example, are actually unhealthful.) Having created this model, I will evaluate common foods and construct meals that are both healthful and thinness promoting. Finally, I will show readers recipes that that are easy to follow and delicious. Thin and healthy - who could ask for more?

Getting back to the triathlon story. When I relayed my Vineman adventures to some friends who were in the race, they said that they were glad I enjoyed my job to which I replied, "What's not to like?"

Well, as they explained, "There are no port-a-potties on the swim portion of the race."

For a moment I was confused, then, in a moment of clarity I said, "Are you saying that all that liquid coming out from their wetsuits wasn't water?"

They just looked at me and smiled.

Chapter 2

YOU AREN'T FAT – YOU JUST NEED TO BE TALLER

When we think about the ideal human image, the sculpture of 'David' by Michelangelo comes to mind. Some would say that this statue represents a "perfectly" proportioned male figure. Wouldn't it be nice if we were all so well constructed? And, if David were human at 14 feet tall, he would certainly be an impressive fellow. However, since he weighs in at 8.5 tons, Michelangelo's David would also be a bit of heavy weight.

Of course, most of us are not made of marble, but rather of more malleable stuff. It is because you and I are malleable, that we are able to change our shapes. Indeed, if you kept the same proportions that you had when you were born, you would be a pretty interesting looking individual. Your head would be the size of a laundry basket and your legs would look like fire hydrants. Not quite the "ideal" form. While we spend most of our youth literally growing "up" into adulthood, our problems start when we stop grow vertically and start growing "out." The challenge is how to keep our growth focused on "taller" and not "wider."

What is the ideal height-to-weight ratio for humans in the 21st century? Many scientists have attempted to answer this question. One

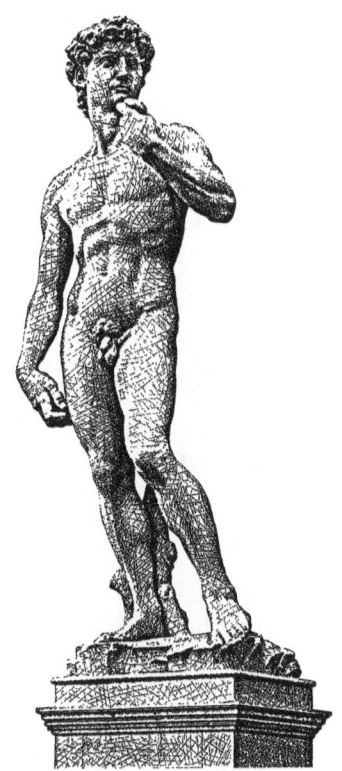

Michelangelo's David

of the first to tackle this problem was a Belgian statistician, named Adolphe Quetelet. He is thought to be the originator of the first Body Mass Index (BMI) scale. Being a very humble fellow, he called his scale the Quetelet Index of Obesity. His formula measured "obesity" by dividing a person's weight (in kilograms) by the square of his or her height (in meters). The advantage of this formula is that it is relatively simple and easy to calculate. Indeed, because it is so simple to use, it has become almost an international standard for calculating the variations from an idealized human height to weight.

$$BMI = W/H^2$$

Say you were a female weighing 125 lbs and 5'7" tall. This would translate into a weight of 56.8 kilos and height of 1.7 meters and that would give a BMI ratio of 19.7. Or, say you are a male who weighs 220 lbs and is 6'0" tall. This individual's ratio would be 27.1. In reviewing typical heights and weights, and looking at the morbidity resulting from these ratios, the scientific community has determined the healthfulness of various values. For those with BMI ratios of less than 18.5, they are deemed as underweight for their height, for those whose BMI are from 18.5 to 25 they are deemed as having a healthy height-to-weight ratio. Moving up the scale, those who have a BMI from 25 to 30 are overweight and those above 30 are obese. You can do this calculation yourself to see where you might fall on this chart. However, this is not the whole story.

While I am sure that lots of well-intentioned folks in the scientific community worked hard to sell the public on the BMI metric, in my view, they appear to have focused on the wrong measurement, body mass. Instead of mass, the calculations, chart, and indeed, the whole focus should be on an individual's height. For example, if we recast BMI in to a Body Height Index (BHI) chart, we arrive at a very different place than the traditional chart. Since we use the same formula as BMI, the values are the same, but the implications are strikingly different.

Like the BMI chart, the BHI chart shows multiple ranges of ratios for individuals. However, unlike BMI, the BHI chart doesn't use any ego crushing words like "fat," "obese" or "overweight" and certainly no name-calling like "unhealthy" or "couch potato." No, at Skinny Foods our approach is all about affirming who you are; and who you are is probably just fine.

Body Height Index

Height →
Weight →

Weight	5'0"	5'1"	5'2"	5'3"	5'4"	5'5"	5'6"	5'7"	5'8"	5'9"	5'10"	5'11"	6'0"	6'1"	6'2"	6'3"	6'4"	6'5"	6'6"	6'7"	6'8"	6'9"	6'10"	6'11"	7'0"	7'1"	7'2"	7'3"	7'4"
120	23.5	22.8	22.0	21.3	20.7	20.0	19.4	18.9	18.3	17.8	17.3	16.8	16.3	15.9	15.5	15.1	14.7	14.3	13.9	13.6	13.2	12.9	12.6	12.3	12.0	11.7	11.4	11.2	10.9
130	25.5	24.7	23.9	23.1	22.4	21.7	21.1	20.4	19.8	19.3	18.7	18.2	17.7	17.2	16.8	16.3	15.9	15.5	15.1	14.7	14.3	14.0	13.6	13.3	13.0	12.7	12.4	12.1	11.8
140	27.4	26.5	25.7	24.9	24.1	23.4	22.7	22.0	21.4	20.7	20.2	19.6	19.1	18.5	18.0	17.6	17.1	16.7	16.2	15.8	15.4	15.1	14.7	14.3	14.0	13.7	13.4	13.1	12.8
150	29.4	28.4	27.5	26.7	25.8	25.1	24.4	23.7	22.9	22.2	21.6	21.0	20.4	19.9	19.3	18.8	18.3	17.9	17.4	17.0	16.5	16.1	15.7	15.3	15.0	14.6	14.3	14.0	13.7
160	31.4	30.3	29.4	28.4	27.5	26.7	25.9	25.2	24.4	23.7	23.0	22.4	21.8	21.2	20.6	20.1	19.5	19.0	18.6	18.1	17.6	17.2	16.8	16.3	16.0	15.6	15.2	14.9	14.6
170	33.3	32.2	31.2	30.2	29.3	28.4	27.5	26.7	25.9	25.2	24.5	23.8	23.1	22.5	21.9	21.3	20.8	20.2	19.7	19.2	18.7	18.3	17.8	17.4	17.0	16.6	16.2	15.8	15.5
180	35.3	34.1	33.0	32.0	31.0	30.1	29.2	28.3	27.5	26.7	25.9	25.2	24.5	23.8	23.2	22.6	21.9	21.4	20.9	20.4	19.8	19.4	18.9	18.4	18.0	17.6	17.2	16.8	16.4
190	37.2	36.0	34.9	33.8	32.7	31.7	30.8	29.9	29.0	28.2	27.4	26.6	25.9	25.2	24.5	23.8	23.2	22.6	22.0	21.5	21.0	20.4	19.9	19.5	19.0	18.6	18.1	17.7	17.3
200	39.2	38.0	36.7	35.6	34.5	33.4	32.4	31.4	30.5	29.6	28.8	28.0	27.2	26.5	25.8	25.1	24.5	23.8	23.2	22.6	22.0	21.5	21.0	20.5	20.0	19.5	19.1	18.7	18.2
210	41.2	39.8	38.5	37.3	36.2	35.1	34.0	33.0	32.1	31.1	30.3	29.4	28.6	27.8	27.1	26.4	25.7	25.0	24.4	23.8	23.2	22.6	22.0	21.5	21.0	20.5	20.0	19.6	19.1
220	43.1	41.7	40.4	39.1	37.9	36.8	35.7	34.6	33.6	32.6	31.7	30.8	30.0	29.1	28.4	27.6	26.9	26.2	25.5	24.9	24.3	23.7	23.1	22.5	22.0	21.5	21.0	20.5	20.1
230	45.1	43.6	42.2	40.9	39.6	38.4	37.3	36.2	35.1	34.1	33.1	32.2	31.3	30.5	29.7	28.9	28.1	27.4	26.7	26.0	25.4	24.7	24.1	23.6	23.0	22.5	22.0	21.5	21.0
240	47.0	45.5	44.1	42.7	41.4	40.1	38.9	37.7	36.6	35.6	34.6	33.6	32.7	31.8	30.9	30.1	29.3	28.6	27.8	27.1	26.5	25.8	25.2	24.6	24.0	23.5	22.9	22.4	21.9
250	49.0	47.4	45.9	44.5	43.1	41.8	40.5	39.3	38.2	37.1	36.0	35.0	34.0	33.1	32.2	31.4	30.6	29.8	29.0	28.3	27.6	26.9	26.3	25.6	25.0	24.4	23.9	23.3	22.8
260	51.0	49.3	47.7	46.2	44.8	43.4	42.1	40.9	39.7	38.5	37.4	36.4	35.4	34.4	33.5	32.6	31.8	30.9	30.2	29.4	28.7	28.0	27.3	26.6	26.0	25.4	24.8	24.2	23.7
270	52.9	51.2	49.6	48.0	46.5	45.1	43.7	42.4	41.2	40.0	38.9	37.8	36.8	35.8	34.8	33.9	33.0	32.1	31.3	30.5	29.8	29.0	28.3	27.7	27.0	26.4	25.8	25.2	24.6
280	54.9	53.1	51.4	49.8	48.2	46.8	45.4	44.0	42.7	41.5	40.3	39.2	38.1	37.1	36.1	35.1	34.2	33.3	32.5	31.7	30.9	30.1	29.4	28.7	28.0	27.3	26.7	26.1	25.5
290	56.8	55.0	53.2	51.6	49.9	48.4	47.0	45.6	44.3	43.0	41.8	40.6	39.5	38.4	37.4	36.4	35.4	34.5	33.6	32.8	32.0	31.2	30.4	29.7	29.0	28.3	27.7	27.0	26.4
300	58.8	56.9	55.1	53.3	51.7	50.1	48.6	47.2	45.8	44.5	43.2	42.0	40.8	39.7	38.7	37.6	36.6	35.7	34.8	33.9	33.1	32.3	31.5	30.7	30.0	29.3	28.6	28.0	27.3

Region labels overlaid on the chart: **Just Right** · **A Little Too Short** · **Way Too Short**

Table 1 - What more do you need to know?

If the calculations show that your BHI ratio is above 32, all it means is that you are "way too short." If your ratio is below 21 you are "just right" and if your ratio is somewhere between 21 and 32 you are just "a little too short." There is nothing wrong with being a bit short. No one gives you dirty looks because you are too short. Your shortness is not from a lack of will power or the fact that you have no self-control around a bowl of Halloween candy, it is just the way you are. But if you want to move down the BHI scale and reveal the thin svelte you that lies beneath those fat corpuscles, maybe all you need to do is increase your height.

Increasing Your Height

When confronting a challenging, technical problem such as how to increase your height, it is often best to start from first principles (the beginning). In the case of humans, and indeed for all mammals, the beginning starts at the moment of conception. For most of us, the Deoxyribonucleic Acid (DNA) that determines our ultimate height is established when your father's sperm meets your mother's egg. Your DNA is a gift from your parents and it is wrapped up in a very small and very pretty little package (your genes).

Throughout your life you get to open the package and see what is inside. Your DNA largely determines your athletic ability, looks, musical talents, and intellect. Your parents may not be fully aware of the choices they made on your behalf, but none-the-less, they provide the stuff that makes you "you."

And, if you don't like who you are, blame your parents. If you are not pretty enough, smart enough, having trouble with addiction or gambling or overeating, it is largely your parents fault. After all, Mom chose Dad and that was the beginning of "you." If she wanted you to be smarter or better looking she should have chosen a smarter or better- looking sperm donor. The same is true with your height as well, if she wanted you to be taller, she should have chosen a taller partner.

As it turns out, lots of women have thought about this and seem to prefer men who are taller than average. Unless you are an incredibly overpaid actor, being tall helps with the ladies. In fact, there is a story about a well-known NBA player who allegedly bedded over 20,000 women. It is not clear if they wanted to have taller children or just a memorable night out, but maybe their sub-conscious mind wanted to give their eggs the best chance to become a tall child. While your DNA is not your destiny, it is a pretty good indicator of who and what you will become.

Therefore, the first step in becoming the slim fit individual is to choose slim-fit parents. If you are reading this, it may be a bit late for you as you are already "whole" from a DNA perspective. However, in the not too distant future, it may be entirely possible to use genetic engineering to modify your DNA to create a different "you." If you want to have blond hair then possibly science could modify your genes to make those brunette follicles produce blonde hair. For those of you who know individuals who are slim and trim but have overweight parents, you may say that weight is not directly heritable (something you inherit from your parents). However, if there is a significant difference between your physique and that of your parent then you might want to get a paternity test. After all, moms are not always the saints that they seem to be. And if your vertical jump is over 40 inches, you might want to ask your mom if she ever dated any basketball players. Yes, picking the right parents is the first and probably the best way to become "David" sans the marble.

Other Methods

Beyond the art of picking better parents, there are a number of other ways to increase one's height. Of course, the first thing that comes to mind is the "rack." Now the rack has a somewhat negative reputation; being primarily a torture device used to elicit confessions. However, the science and engineering behind the rack is sound, even if its original purpose is painfully brutal. Basically, practitioners of this devise were applying a force on a system to try and elongate it. Now, for systems that are highly malleable such as a rubber band, stretching it does increase its length while reducing its waist size (so to speak).

Unfortunately, for those who had the experience firsthand, the human body isn't so malleable and rapid stretching was purposefully painful. In those cases the stretching was done too quickly to be effective at increasing an individual's height. However, if the stretching was done more slowly, giving the body a chance to adjust to the applied force, then the limbs would have grown longer and the spine stretched.

Unlikely, you say? Well, this is the exact principle behind orthodontia. When braces are put on an individual's teeth they are applying a force to move the teeth to a more cosmetically appealing or efficient position. Since teeth are firmly rooted in bone the process takes many months. But move they do, as the body adjusts to the applied force.

If the rack isn't your thing, then you might try the 20th century version of the rack, gravity boots. In this case, gravity is the applying force and hanging upside down for an extended period of time allows gravity to do the work. Cheap and reliable, gravity pulls down on all your constituent parts and allows them to adjust to the force. Your spine will decompress as the disks are allowed to refill with fluid. The same is true with your other joints. Even a brief time hanging time upside down will allow you to regain some of the height you lost due to constant exposure to downward gravity.

You might ask, "How long would I have to hang upside down to make these changes permanent?" Great question, but the answer is probably longer than you would want. Humans weren't constructed to be upside down for extended periods of time. For one thing the blood vessels (veins) in our body have valves that help push blood back to our heart. For veins to function properly they need to be compressed and that is where walking and exercise come in. As long as you are moving you are alternatively compressing and releasing veins which causes your blood to move along. Unfortunately, hanging upside down is a pretty stationary endeavor and will only lead to a major headache as your skull fills with fluid.

Speaking of gravity, another tried and true method to increase your height is space travel. Studies have shown that astronauts can be as much as 2 inches taller, after just a few weeks in space. The reason for their increased height is that the gravity that you and I normally experience is not pressing down on space travelers. Similar to gravity boots, the effect is due to increased space in the cartilage between vertebrae in our spines. Take the weight off and you will become taller.

If you want to see this effect for yourself, measure your height before you go to bed (when you will be the shortest), and when you rise (when you will be the tallest), and you should see a difference. However, without having to work against the constant pull of gravity, humans rapidly lose their musculature and will become exhausted at almost any exertion.

Early Russian Cosmonauts, in orbit for many months, often had to be carried out of their capsules when they returned to earth. Plus, there is the cost of being launched into space atop a very expensive and somewhat unreliable rocket. Unfortunately, space travel while exciting, and possibly relaxing, is not a very practical way to gain a few inches.

Why not try chemical means to gain height? After all, there seems to be a drug for everything, so why not one to increase one's height? As it turns out, the drug that seems to offer the best result is human growth hormone (HGH). This is the same one that many athletes take to increase their muscle mass, and regain their youthful vigor and flexibility. When first discovered, HGH was thought to be a wonder drug. It was going to be a fountain of youth for all adults, keeping your body young, even if your mind continued to age. And for many folks, it does have that effect. However, like most drugs, use of HGH can come with unwanted side effects. The typical side effects for HGH include the growth of the brow and jaw. Long-term use often brings on joint pain and an increased risk of some types of cancer. Not a pretty picture, but if you can get a prescription for the drug it might be worth a try.

The Top Line

While you are working on increasing your height, you might as well do something about the other part of the equation: your body mass. At Skinny Foods, we work both sides of the equation, and for some, it may be easier to reduce your weight than increase your height. Given a predetermined set of genes, diet plays a significant role in your overall body shape. We, at Skinny Food, have developed an effective approach to addressing the diet issue, one that will give you the body shape that you desire.

Chapter 3

THE SCIENCE BEHIND THE SKINNY FOOD DIET OR THE "THEORY OF THIN"

The Theory of Thin

The Theory of Thin is based on a simple proposition: eating thin foods will help you to become thin. Hard to believe, but true. If you think about the foods that are unhealthy, they are invariably man-made and shaped as spheres or near spheres (i.e. cubes) such as cupcakes, donuts, hamburgers, mashed potatoes, and lasagna. While eating these foods satisfy your hunger for most of us, their high energy density (i.e. calories) lead to weight gain and the host of problems that accompany the "few extra" pounds.

To lose those extra pounds, many folks try diets that offer prepackaged foods or strict limits on how much you can eat. These types of diets are simple, and easy to think about, but hard to do. What happens when you have that mid-afternoon sugar lull or want to eat a second helping? Other diets offer quick fixes, via smoothies, shakes or high fat/high protein foods. And these diets ultimately fail because they are short-term approaches to calorie intake, and don't offer a long-term eating strategy. No, the answer is to find a simple healthy diet; one that allows you to eat all you want while reinforcing the image of what you want to become - thin.

Some of you may think that eating thin foods to become thin is too simplistic and can't possibly work. I know how you feel, and for a time, I felt the same way myself, sharing in your skepticism. But what I found is that foods in their natural state that are long, thin are generally lower in calories, with more fiber and more nutrients than food with spherical shapes. Think about nuts, spherical or near spheres all of them, how about rice or beans or peas, ditto.

Many fruits follow the same pattern, high in calories and low in nutrients. Interesting, the same pattern holds true for many man-made foods such as cakes, pies, and snack foods. Manufacturers are in the business of producing unhealthy foods that are physically compact. Why, might you ask? The answer is simply to reduce packaging and shipping costs. No rocket science here - it is all about the profits. Of course, there are a few exceptions, potato chips for one, are packaged in a large voluminous bags. Mostly air, but at least it somewhat resembles the original ingredient. However, even here, manufactures have worked to "re-optimize" the potato chip via a new production process; eliminating the whole potato in favor of potato flour and corn starch producing stackable chips.

The Formula

As we will see, the Theory of Thin which started out as a simple premise has enormous implications. And like all good scientific theories, there is often an equation or two that explains the principle elements of the theory. When I was completing my undergraduate education, one of my professors commented that although he had done a large body of work on structural dynamics, and had written many papers on the subject, the scientific community remembered him for a small, short equation,. I suspect that Einstein felt the same way when the public boiled down special relativity to just $E=mc^2$ and so too, it is with the Theory of Thin. All of the calculations and analysis come down to the following:

$$FHI_{personal} = Lo^{Se}/(W_{eig}*H*T)$$

FHI - Food Health Index
Lo - Length
SE - Synthetic Effect
Weig - Width
H - Height
T - Body Type

With careful inspection, readers will see that on the left-hand side of the equal sign creates a new measure for food healthfulness, the Food Health Index (**FHI**). The FHI is a measure of the goodness of a food based on a number of input parameters, such as the food's length, width, height, and whether it is natural or synthetic (man-made). The FHI is also influenced by the dieter's body type and their previous experience with diets. At the risk of over simplifying the Theory of Thin, foods with higher values of FHI are better.

To put this into perspective, values from 0 to 1 are uniformly bad and foods scoring in this range must be avoided. Values from 1 to 10 are not quite so bad and may be consumed in limited quantity. Values from 10 to 100 are beneficial foods and may be consumed as part of your daily diet. While values above 100 are skinny super foods and can be consumed anytime and anywhere; breakfast, lunch, dinner, or as a late-night snack. Those who faithfully practice the Skinny Food Diet are not hungry.

It is important to note that FHI is specific for an individual depending on their particular input parameters. For some individuals, there will be foods that score well for them, but poorly for their friends and family. Chapter 5 offers a list of foods and their FHI for a variety of body types. Many readers will be shocked to learn that their beloved apple or pear or even favorite cereals don't score well on the FHI scale. I share in your loss. I too, had to give up some of my treasured foods, but you will be stronger and thinner for having taken the first step of recognizing unhealthy foods. Now with the FHI in mind, we can begin to approach the rest of the Theory of Thin.

Readers will see that the first term to the right of the equal sign (the numerator) is the length of the food. As FHI is non-dimensional, the Length (**Lo**) can be measured in any unit - (they will divide out when the equation is completed.) The **Lo** is then raised to a higher power via the Synthetic Effect (**Se**) based on whether it exists in its natural form ([2]), or to a lower power ([1]), if it was modified through a man-made process. As higher FHIs are better, this argues that foods that are long and natural are preferable to those that are short and man-made.

The first two terms in the denominator are measures of the width (**W**) and height (**H**). Because we are looking for large FHI values, terms in the denominator should be small. First, let us consider cylindrical foods such as hot dogs, spaghetti or pretzels. Because they are cylinders these foods will have equal and relatively small values for their height and width. Consequently, they will have higher FHI scores than other food shapes. Unlike cylinders, foods that are shaped like spheres will have similar measurements for their length, width, and height. These foods do not score well on the FHI scale and should be avoided.

Finally, there are foods shaped like disks including foods such as pancakes, chips or even lettuce. These foods will have very different values for their width and height. In the case of leafy vegetables, the width is large but the height is very small so the product of these two factors is also a small number and these foods will have a relatively high FHI. For most man-maid foods the situation changes significantly. Hamburgers, cupcakes, and donuts have a significant thickness and when the thickness is multiplied by the width, the unhealthfulness of these foods becomes readily apparent. A large denominator either in the case of the USDA food pyramid or on your body is a bad thing.

Body Types and Dieting History

Readers will further note that the Theory of Thin equation includes a term (**T**) combining your dieting history with body type. In a number of ways, these terms are linked. For example, people with certain body types (endomorphic) typically have a great deal of difficulty losing weight and may have tried multiple diets; often with little success. While others with the slender body type (ectomorphic) may never have needed to diet, and those with the mesomorphic body type, are someplace in between. While this seems simple enough, for those that have tried multiple diets, there may be an additional factor at work: "diet hysteresis."

In scientific terms, hysteresis is a phenomenon whereas the outcome of an event is determined in some part based on prior history. For example, consider a coin flip. There is no hysteresis in this system because whether the coin lands heads or tail has nothing to with the prior flips. On the other hand, a system with hysteresis may be your ability to achieve good results from your weight loss diet. Research on dieting has shown this "yo-yo" effect. You lose weight but gain it back and the second time you try to lose weight find it is harder to lose the same pounds you lost before, and so on. It is almost like your body is preparing for future cycles of famine and plenty and makes sure that you store up fat for the pending famine.

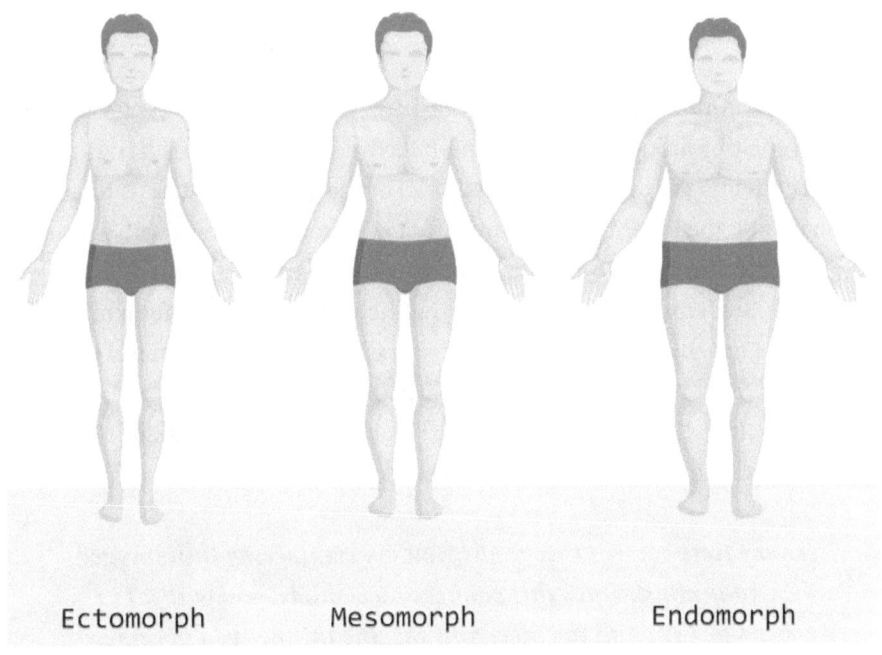

Ectomorph   Mesomorph   Endomorph

Body Types

Let us then consider elements of the T-factor. If you have an ectomorphic body type and you never dieted then your T-factor is 1. (Recall that low numbers in the denominator are good). On the other hand, if you are an endomorphic individual and you have tried every diet under the sun, then your T-factor score is a 3. The T-factor also helps explain why some folks can each pretty much anything they want and not gain an ounce. It helps quantize this effect, and as we shall see in later chapters, folks with higher T- factors will invariably have different FHI scores for the same food than folks with lower T-factors.

The Skinny Food Diet is the first diet that makes this distinction. Recognizing these differences makes the Skinny Food Diet measurably more successful than others. And whether it is in your DNA, your metabolic rate or simply your lifestyle, customizing the diet to those differences is a key part of the Skinny Food approach. The primary equation behind the Theory of Thin is simple, robust, and uncomplicated. By now, some readers are ready to move on and start the diet. We applaud your enthusiasm and suggest that you go directly to chapter 4 and see what foods are right for you.

Physiological Component

However, before we leave the Theory of Thin, we would be remiss if we didn't address the physiology behind the diet. An important part of changing personal behavior is to create a mental model of the behavior we hope to create. If you want to be nicer then you must first envision nice behavior. Similarly, if you wish to be thin, you need to see yourself as thin.

There is a famous public speaker that helps people become rich. Part of his pitch is to tell people that they are already millionaires, even if they are broke. You have to see it first and then you can create it. So, too, it is with becoming thin. If you see yourself as thin, you are half way there. And that is where the Skinny Food Diet comes in to play.

Every time you eat thin foods, you are reinforcing thin images in your mind. Once this connection is made, you will eat to become thin and the more you eat, the thinner you become.

Special Cases

Finally, we need to address foods that are not of any particular shape, and these are liquids. With the exception of water most, all other liquids are man-made and generally should be avoided. Juices, soda, beer, wine, and the like are loaded with calories and are unhealthful. Some liquids, like milk and juice, are more natural, but here again, are made or modified by man. Pasteurized, homogenized, bottled or canned; these are all produced in ways that run counter to the skinny food approach.

We recommend against consuming these liquids. However, if you find that you can't imagine how you will get through the day without a banana, wheat grass smoothie, we have a Skinny Food solution for you. Drink your smoothie or any beverage you choose through a straw. Yes, a straw! Research has shown that by sucking beverages through a straw confers the benefits of the Skinny Food Diet to your liquid of choice. In fact, the smaller the diameter of the straw is, the greater the benefit. Wine, beer, vodka shots, juice, whatever you are consuming, can all be improved with a small diameter straw. Adding an umbrella to the drink couldn't hurt either.

Other foods such as oils, sauces, and condiments are really blobs (spheres). Not much good to say about theses food items. Food companies developed most of these foods in laboratories for the sole purpose of getting rid of surplus commodities. These foods generally follow the same pattern; thick, gelatinous, quivering blobs of fat, starch, salt and artificial flavors. Whatever they are, they are not good for you. Avoid them as best you can.

And then there is water. Water is necessary for life itself and we can't live without it. Turns out that nature has provided the answer to this question of what to drink. In some climates, we find water frozen into a solid state and it is here that we find the solution to the liquid conforming to the Skinny Food mantra. Icicles: yes, icicles. Mother nature created the perfect Skinny Food drink, and all you have to do is heat and serve.

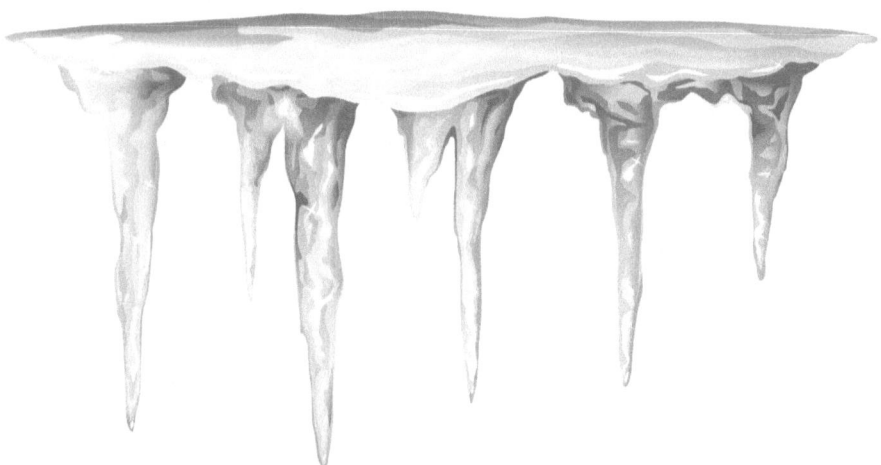

Icicles - Your daily water supply

Chapter 4

ARE YOU RIGHT FOR THE SKINNY FOOD DIET?

By now, you are probably thinking that the Skinny Food Diet is just what I have been looking for: a simple plan that is easy to follow with delicious foods. And you would be right. It is a simple plan and one that guarantees results. However, not everyone is accepted into the Skinny Food Diet "club." There are some folks who, for often reasons beyond their control, are just not worthy. They may not have the right disposition, temperament, lack willpower or are unable to remember basic instructions. They could also be people who cannot do simple addition, subtraction or the dreaded division. Finally, they could be folks who are so in love with their current diet plan, that they are unable to recognize something better when it comes along.

If you do not fall into any of these obviously negative categories, I devised a simple test to see if you are right for the Skinny Food Diet. The following is a list of 10 questions. Answer them as best can.

Skinny Food Diet Suitability Quiz

1) When you look in the mirror what do you see?
    a) A thin person trapped in a fat person's body
    b) A person who needs to lose a few pounds
    c) Someone who is in good shape
    d) A god or goddess

2) When you were young, were you made fun of because of which of the following?
   a) You had big feet
   b) You had big ears
   c) You wore glasses
   d) You were the one making fun of everybody else

3) When you think about diets, you do which of the following?
   a) Get nervous
   b) Get excited
   c) Get hungry
   d) Get ready to cheat

4) You dream about which of the following?
   a) Food
   b) Puppies
   c) Sex
   d) Nothing

5) How many thin friends do you have?
   a) None
   b) A few
   c) A lot
   d) Everyone I know is thin

6) When you are sad, you do which of the following?
   a) Eat
   b) Watch old movies
   c) Fall asleep
   d) Cry

7) You live in which of the following type of home?
   a) Flat
   b) Townhouse
   c) Walk-up apartment
   d) Country house

8) You like to go grocery shopping when you are which of the following?
    a) Hungry
    b) Full
    c) A bit hung over
    d) My spouse does all the shopping

9) You can follow simple instructions when?
    a) All the time
    b) Some of the time
    c) Not so much
    d) Almost never

10) When you hear the phrase "Hey, Skinny," you do which of the following?
    a) Blush
    b) Get mad
    c) Think they are talking about someone else
    d) Turn around, smile, and say "thank you"

Scoring - for each "A" give yourself four points, for each "B" three points, each "C" two points and each "D" one point. Give yourself an additional 2 points for each odd numbered question you answered with the letter "B" and 1 point for each even number question you answered "C." Add up your score. The next part is a bit tricky, take the square root of your age rounding down to nearest whole number and add it to the total. The resultant number is your SFDSS (**S**kinny **F**ood **D**iet **S**uitability **S**core).

Results

Negative Numbers - If you calculated a negative number, you are not a good candidate for the Skinny Food Diet. And it's not because you don't have the right body type or lack willpower. No, if you got a negative SFDSS it means that you lack basic math skills and frankly your time could be better spent in remedial algebra.

Zero - If you came up with zero, you probably gave up too early. Unfortunately for some, this can be a lifelong pattern; they just can't commit. Think about the original Beatle's drummer Pete Best. In 1962, he decided that the band wasn't going anywhere and left the group only to be replaced by Ringo Starr. (Actually, he was fired, but the story is so much better told the other way round).

Positive Numbers – Congratulations! You are perfect for the Skinny Food Diet. Not only can you do higher math, but also you have the stick-to-it attitude, that is so lacking in modern society. If you are ready, read on because it's time to get serious about Skinny Foods.

Chapter 5

FINDING YOUR PERFECT SKINNY FOODS

"Water, water everywhere and not a drop to drink." At Skinny Foods, we know exactly how the Ancient Mariner must have felt as he lay dying of thirst, adrift in an ocean surrounded by salt water (Rime of the Ancient Marnier, Coleridge 1798). Before modern survival equipment, being lost at sea was a struggle that only a few would survive. The waves, sun, dehydration, hypothermia, and starvation would all take their toll on unfortunate sailors. And, if you ended up in a life raft without supplies, many a sailor would in desperation try to drink salt water, only to vomit it back up. The sailor's stomach reacted to the high concentration of salt with a powerful and involuntary act, eliminating it as quickly as possible.

Yes, even though we are surrounded by the 'land of plenty' the foods we are given are as unpalatable as salt water was to the Mariner. Imagine how interesting life would be if your body had a similar reaction to a half-pound cheeseburger as it did to salt water. "Drive through" would take on a whole new meaning as your lower gastrointestinal tract sought to eliminate unhealthy foods. No, the challenge we face is one of making healthy food choices. In a perfect world, where only skinny foods are available, Homer Simpson's version of this quote might be more apt, "Water, water everywhere, so let's all have a drink."

Unfortunately for Homer, beer is not on the Skinny Food diet. However, let's take a look at the types of foods that are on the diet, ones that are thin and healthy and can become a part of your everyday diet. Our Chapter 3 calculations showed us that we are seeking natural foods that are long in one dimension and short in the other two. Cylinders and long rectangles are the optimum shapes for our Super Skinny Foods. The best of the best, spaghetti and breadsticks instantly come to mind, vegetables such as green beans, asparagus, zucchini, and fruits like bananas, and candies like licorice. And of course we can't forget everybody's favorite - French fries. A "guilty pleasure" perhaps, but at Skinny Foods we don't judge. We are all about leading the way to thinness and if French fries are your thing, who are we to say no?

Back To Body Types

Before jumping into the calculations and charts, recall from Chapter 3 that the Skinny Food model is tailored to your particular body type. If you are one of the lucky ones who have an ectomorphic body, you can probably eat whatever you want, and not gain much weight. Good for you. However, the Skinny Food diet is still important, as it is the only diet using formulas and calculations to create the "just right for you" approach to healthy eating. No more guess work, no more "should I or shouldn't I" confusion. No, the answer to the question of what to eat is straightforward and simple, follow the chart and your health will be assured.

Now if you are a mesomorphic, body type, you generally have to watch what you are eating. You might find that after the holidays, you have put on a few pounds. Health club memberships are sold to the mesomorphic folks. They are the ones who can easily build muscle, lose a few inches and look good doing it. For you, the Skinny Food Diet will help make you look and feel better. And when you are completing your 1-hour workout on the Stair Master, just make sure to tell the folks at the gym that your skinny new body is due to the Skinny Food Diet.

If, on the other hand, you happen to have an endomorphic body type, you are most always on a diet or, at least, thinking about dieting. It is for you, the Skinny Food Diet was created. No more having to think about what to eat. No more counting calories, no more measuring grams of fat or protein and certainly none of those annoying Paleo digestion problems. No, at Skinny Foods we are all about healthy eating, using nature to guide your food decisions. Nature has already determined which foods are healthful just look at their shape.

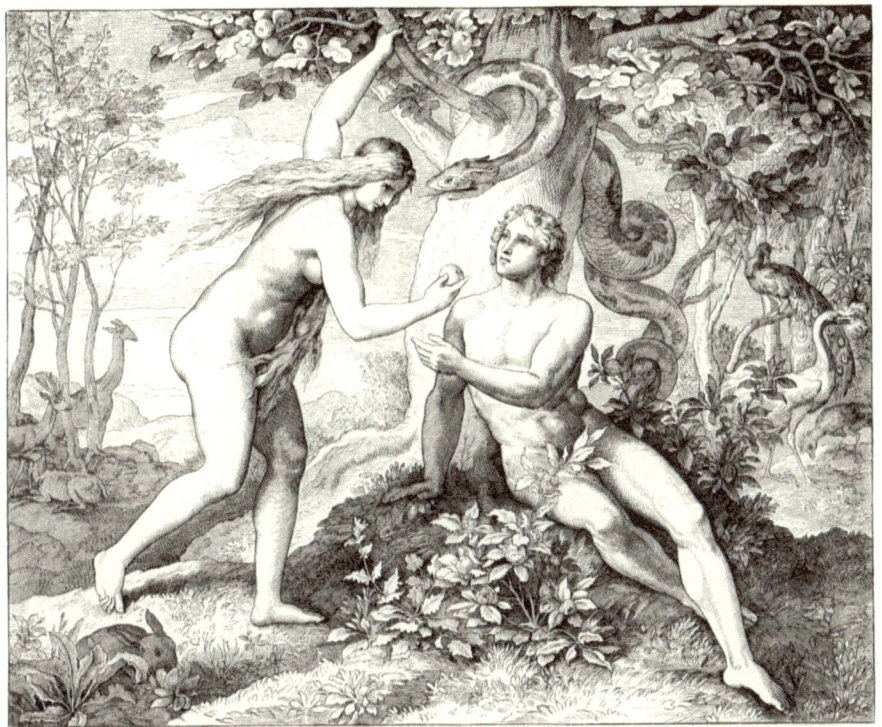

Adam and Eve and the Snake

After all, Adam and Eve were not kicked out of the Garden of Eden for eating a carrot, stalk of celery or green bean (high FHIs). No, it was for eating an apple (low FHI). And to carry this thought just a step further, if they had eaten the snake (probably a Skinny Super Food with an FHI well above 100) instead of the apple, they wouldn't have been in trouble in the first place. Like Mr. Simpson, Adam and Eve didn't know about the Skinny Food diet. If they had, human history might have been far different. But they had to learn the hard way. Fortunately, you can learn from their mistakes.

FHI Calculations

Let's look at some calculations for popular foods, starting with the super skinny food, spaghetti. Uncooked spaghetti is a long smooth cylinder about 12 inches long and about ⅛ inch high and ⅛ inch wide. Cooked spaghetti is just about as long, but swells as it absorbs water and becomes about $\frac{3}{16}$ inch high and $\frac{3}{16}$ inch wide.

Since very few people eat uncooked spaghetti, let's use the cooked dimensions. First, if we convert our fractions to decimals, $\frac{3}{16}$'s becomes 0.1875. Next, we need to determine our body type. Personally, I am a mix of all types, but am closest overall to a Mesomorphic type or a "2." Finally, we need to note that spaghetti is a man-made food, so it gets a "1" for its' synthetic effect. Now we can put these values into the FHI formula.

$$FHI = 12^{(1)}/(0.1875*0.1875*2)$$
$$FHI = 170.7$$

With a score over 100, spaghetti is a super skinny food. So, grab a big bowl of your favorite and dig in.

How about a cucumber? Its length is about 10 inches and is a natural product, so the synthetic effect is a 2. Its height and width are both about 2 inches, and again, using my mesomorphic body type, the factor is 2.

$$FHI = 10^{(2)}/(2*2*2)$$
$$FHI = 12.5$$
A good wholesome skinny food

Let's do a similar calculation for a hot dog. The length is about 6 inches, it is clearly a man-made product so the synthetic effect is 1, the width is about 1-inch the height is also 1- inch and again we are using the mesomorphic body type of 2. So the FHI for a hot dog is:

$$FHI = 6^{(1)}/(1*1*2)$$
$$FHI = 3.0$$

Not a great food, consumption should be limited. But if you want to have a hot dog with your green beans, that's OK.

Descending into food hell, we come to the short, fat foods. There are plenty to choose from, but let's look at the lowly meatball. It is more or less a perfect sphere so let's assume that it is 2.0" in length, width and height. It is man-made (Se = 1) and using my body type of 2 we have the following:

$$FHI = 2.0^{(1)}/(2.0*2.0*2)$$
$$FHI = 0.25$$

With a value less than 1, meatballs and all other foods like them should be avoided.

To save readers from the effort of calculating the FHI for various foods we constructed a table for 99 common foods. Readers who are handy with spreadsheets and/or calculators may want to perform calculations based on your own measurements. And for the thousands of other food items in the marketplace, you will need to come up with your own list. However, at Skinny Foods, we are happy to help. Starting with common foods will give readers a flavor for the types of foods that we are looking for. In fact one of the most beautiful parts of the Skinny Food diet is its ease. You can pretty much just look a food and determine its goodness.

In fact, the diet is so intuitive that a child of 6 can be taught the basics. Let's check in with a neighborhood boy, Bobby Smith. Bobby is a bright fellow with lots of good sense. When explained the basics of the Skinny Food Diet he responded,

"So, if I eat green beans or carrots I will get skinny? That's great because I love green beans and carrots. I like crunchy foods. One time I got a carrot stick stuck in my ....."

Yes, Bobby you've got it. The fundamentals of the Skinny Food Diet are pretty obvious. As soon as your child starts eating solid food, start them out with a banana and they will be committed for life. By becoming a Skinny Food family, you will give you child the gift of thinness, as well as intelligence and popularity, every parent's dream. Get your paper and pencil out and put in some quality time in with your children doing Skinny Food calculations. You will be glad you did.

The first 49 foods, those shown on the chart include a variety of foods ranging from those Skinny Super Foods with FHIs above 100 to those that are marginally acceptable for the Skinny Food diet with an FHI of 1.0. Starting with the top of the list we can all imagine a dinner meal of spaghetti, breadsticks with a kale salad as a Skinny Food winner. Or how about a strip steak fajita meal with spring onions, green chilies, and tortillas? For those who are true meat eaters we have short ribs and steak tacos. And, if you are a pescatarian (eat fish) the Skinny Food diet won't let you down, offering up crab legs, lobster tail, salmon and tilapia filets and trout.

Vegetarians in the group will be pleased with the Skinny Food choices as well. Starting with a number of pasta dishes, Skinny Food selections include spaghetti squash, yams and about 20 choices of vegetables - foods for every palate, temperament, and disposition. And when those late night cravings hit you, open a bag of pretzels or jerky to tide you over till morning.

The second page contains some foods that are healthful and worthy, but many that are not. You will note that many popular foods have an FHI of less than 1. These are foods to avoid. The Skinny Food diet doesn't need to remind readers about the problems with most of the round foods, just look at them. Is this the body shape you want?.

Let's check in with the Smith family and see how the Skinny Food Diet was received.

> **Bobby's Mother, Ms. Smith aged 36** - *"Thanks for explaining this to Bobby. I see how this diet works and it is amazing how simple it is. I like how you show why BMI is not the best way to determine one's ideal height. When you consider diets, the BHI, and the FHI scale make more sense."*

Well done Ms. Smith - you've "got it" as well.

Food Health Index (FHI)

	Skinny Foods	Endomorph	Mesomorph	Ectomorph
1	Spaghetti	113.78	170.67	341.33
2	Kale	106.67	160.00	320.00
3	Jerky	106.67	160.00	320.00
4	String Cheese	85.33	128.00	256.00
5	Asparagus	85.33	128.00	256.00
6	Green Beans	79.37	119.05	238.10
7	Bread Sticks	64.00	96.00	192.00
8	Crab Legs	48.00	72.00	144.00
9	Lettuce	40.00	60.00	120.00
10	Anchovies (canned)	37.50	56.25	112.50
11	Fiber Cereal	33.33	50.00	100.00
12	French Fries	26.67	40.00	80.00
13	Stick Pretzels	25.00	37.50	75.00
14	Sardines (fresh)	24.00	36.00	72.00
15	Carrots	21.33	32.00	64.00
16	Bananas	21.33	32.00	64.00
17	Strip Steak	21.33	32.00	64.00
18	Zucchini	21.33	32.00	64.00
19	Spinach (Fresh)	20.00	30.00	60.00
20	Shrimp	14.81	22.22	44.44
21	Sardines (Canned)	14.22	21.33	42.67
22	Bacon	13.33	20.00	40.00
24	Eggplant	12.00	18.00	36.00
25	Trout	12.00	18.00	36.00
23	Canolli	8.33	12.50	25.00
26	Hot Peppers	8.33	12.50	25.00
27	Cucumbers	8.33	12.50	25.00
28	Egg (Fried)	6.67	10.00	20.00
29	Potato Chip	6.67	10.00	20.00
30	Tilopia	6.00	9.00	18.00
31	Corn (On The Cob)	5.33	8.00	16.00
36	Taquitos	5.33	8.00	16.00
32	Granola Bar	4.27	6.40	12.80
33	Sausage Link	4.00	6.00	12.00
34	Pickles (Dill Spears)	3.56	5.33	10.67
35	Salmon Filet	3.27	4.90	9.80
37	Lobster Tail	2.78	4.17	8.33
38	Grape Nuts	2.67	4.00	8.00
39	Oatmeal	2.67	4.00	8.00
40	Short Ribs	2.67	4.00	8.00
41	Popsicles	2.33	3.50	7.00
42	Granola Bar	2.22	3.33	6.67
43	Hotdog	2.00	3.00	6.00
44	Chocolate Bar	1.67	2.50	5.00
45	Almonds	1.33	2.00	4.00
46	Pancake	1.33	2.00	4.00
47	Baguette	1.33	2.00	4.00
48	M & M's	1.33	2.00	4.00
49	Mini Wheat cereal	1.11	1.67	3.33

Food Health Index (FHI)

Fat Foods		Endomorph	Mesomorph	Ectomorph
50	Pizza (slice)	1.07	1.60	3.20
51	Buffalo Wings	1.00	1.50	3.00
52	Baked Potatoes	0.93	1.39	2.78
53	Toast	0.83	1.25	2.50
54	Sausage Patty	0.83	1.25	2.50
55	Tacos	0.78	1.17	2.33
56	Olives	0.75	1.13	2.25
57	Watermelon	0.75	1.13	2.25
58	Tater tots	0.67	1.00	2.00
59	Shushi (all kinds)	0.67	1.00	2.00
60	Chocolate Chip Cookie	0.67	1.00	2.00
61	Waffles	0.67	1.00	2.00
62	Twinkie	0.59	0.89	1.78
63	Fortune Cookie	0.50	0.75	1.50
64	Oysters	0.50	0.75	1.50
65	Croutons	0.44	0.67	1.33
66	Apple Pie (slice)	0.39	0.58	1.17
67	Hamburger (patty)	0.33	0.50	1.00
68	Peas	0.33	0.50	1.00
69	Broccoli	0.33	0.50	1.00
70	Tomatoes	0.33	0.50	1.00
71	Apple	0.33	0.50	1.00
72	Orange	0.33	0.50	1.00
73	Beets	0.33	0.50	1.00
74	Chicken	0.33	0.50	1.00
75	Cantelope	0.33	0.50	1.00
76	Turkey	0.33	0.50	1.00
77	Ham	0.33	0.50	1.00
78	Popcorn	0.33	0.50	1.00
79	Brownie	0.33	0.50	1.00
80	Strawberries	0.33	0.50	1.00
81	Cheese Burger	0.30	0.44	0.89
82	Burrito	0.22	0.33	0.67
83	Philli Cheese Steak Sandwich	0.22	0.33	0.67
84	Banana Split	0.19	0.28	0.56
85	Meat ball	0.17	0.25	0.50
86	Hard Boiled Egg	0.17	0.25	0.50
87	Donuts	0.17	0.25	0.50
88	Soups (all types)	0.17	0.25	0.50
89	Grits	0.17	0.25	0.50
90	Mac and Cheese	0.17	0.25	0.50
91	Meat Loaf	0.17	0.25	0.50
92	Lasagna	0.13	0.20	0.40
93	Milk (quart carton)	0.13	0.19	0.38
94	Ice Cream (single scoop)	0.11	0.17	0.33
95	Pudding (bowl)	0.11	0.17	0.33
96	Sour Cream (tub)	0.11	0.17	0.33
97	Muffins	0.11	0.17	0.33
98	Nacho Plate	0.08	0.13	0.25
99	Tuna Noodle Cassarole	0.08	0.12	0.23

Chapter 6

SIZE REALLY DOES MATTER

When it comes to the Skinny Food Diet, size really does matter. Recall the scene from the movie, "Animal House." As the wife of Dean Wormer inspects a rather large cucumber, one of the fraternity members approaches and says, "Vegetables can be really sensuous, don't you think?"

The dean's wife reminded him, "Vegetables are sensual - people are sensuous."

What she neglected to say is, "skinny food vegetables and all skinny foods are wonderfully sensual. Some, like this cucumber, are long and hard while others are thick, torrid cylinders bursting with life-giving juices, waiting to be picked, cooked and eaten." Panting slightly she would continue, "Skinny Food is all about creating the body that you desire, long, lean, and hard like a cucumber." Breathing heavily she would finish with, "and that is why we should all be on the Skinny Food Diet." This could have been the way the scene ended, but unfortunately for those at the college, the Skinny Food Diet was not yet discovered. It was too bad for them. However, the story ends well as the fraternity member asks the Dean's wife to a college toga party and the rest is cinematic history.

Shopping for Skinny Foods

As long as we are in the supermarket, let's apply the Skinny Food principles to the rest of our shopping. In the average American supermarket, there are over 50,000 items and lots to look at. And among the 50,000 items, we are likely to find some great skinny foods items. How do you know? Well, in addition to bringing your own shopping bags and a list, an important part of skinny food shopping gear is now a ruler. Yes, a ruler, something to measure the length, width and height of our purchases. Just like Mrs. Wormer, we want to make sure that our purchases are appropriately sized. And since we are in the produce aisle let's see what looks good.

Leeks, spring onions, and zucchini all are winners. Green beans, carrots, celery, and cucumbers certainly meet the Skinny Food test. When we come to the eggplant, we will need to look for the Japanese or Chinese varieties as the regular type are more short and squat. Laying on its side a typical Japanese eggplant is about 9 inches long by 2 inches wide and 2 inches high and with these dimensions has an FHI of 16. Regular eggplant may be as long but are about 5 inches tall and just as wide - its FHI is 3. Both are acceptable, but long and thin is how we want to look so we look for and buy the Asian varieties.

Moving along the aisle we pick up kale, lettuce, spinach, and asparagus. We add the fresh parsley, cilantro, rosemary, and thyme. We can skip the beets, potatoes, onions, turnips, and winter squash, as all are short and squat. One winter squash that we do buy is the spaghetti squash. Once it is cooked, its flesh turns into wondrous strands of flaxen goodness (more on this later). Skip the melons, cantaloupe, honeydew, apples, oranges, pears and plums. Ditto for all the berries. Strawberry, blueberries, raspberries and blackberries are all no-nos. Bananas, on the other hand is a perfect skinny food.

Rounding the corner, we see Ms, Smith.

> **Ms. Smith age 36** - *"Hi neighbor! Fancy running into you in the supermarket - I really appreciate you taking the time to explain the Skinny Food Diet. I am now on the lookout for the best skinny foods. Your chart makes it so easy to find the right foods."*

Ms. Smith, you are right. Because you never know when you will need to make a food decision, I carry my Skinny Food chart, ruler and calculator with me wherever I go.

After the produce section, we both turn to the bakery. Not much to see here but since we are on the hunt for Skinny Foods, we pick up some breadsticks and a baguette. Skip all the cakes, pies, donuts, muffins and bread. Delicious no doubt, but do you really want to look like a bran muffin? Turning the aisle we see on the end cap, a packages of tortillas. Although, they are long and wide, they are also very thin and like spinach and lettuce score a 10 on the FHI scale.

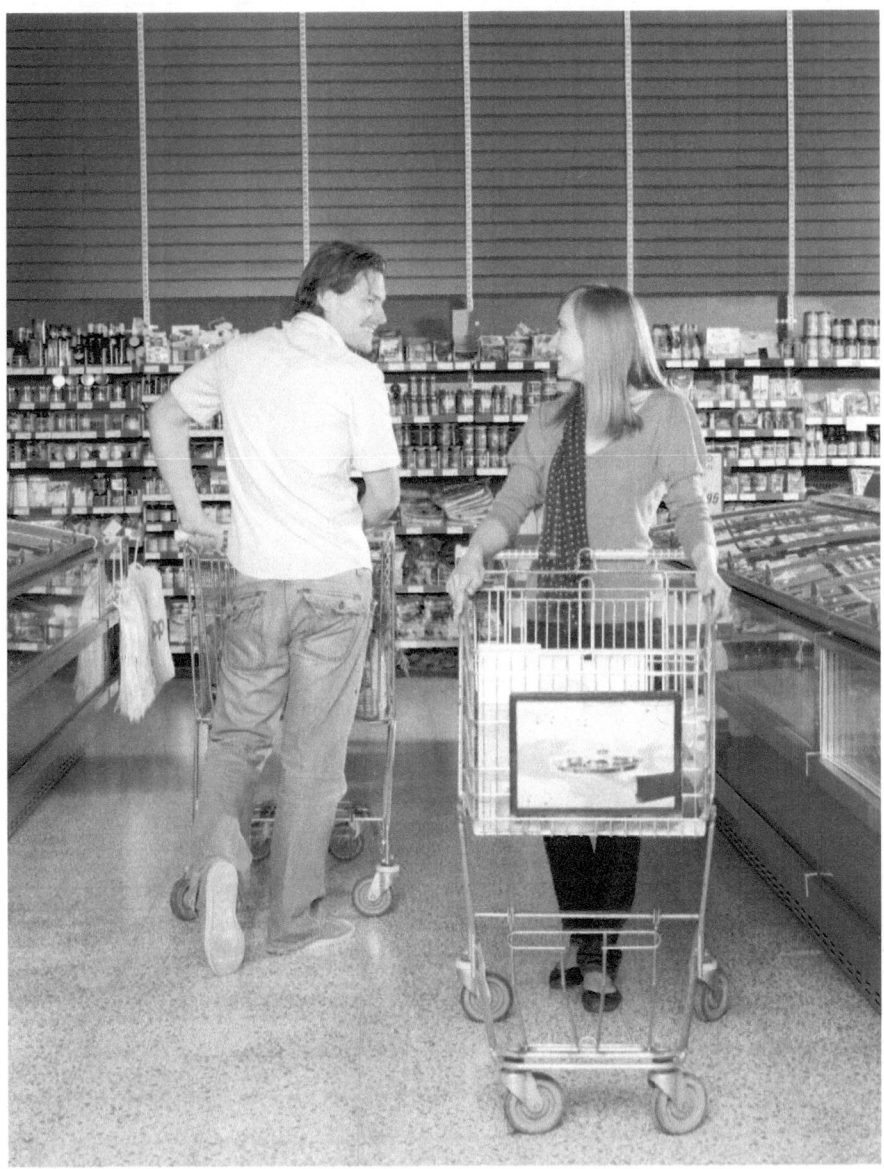

The author meets Ms. Smith shopping for Skinny Foods

As I turn the corner, I find myself heading into the cereal aisle. Here, it is a challenge to find something that meets the Skinny Food model. Let's review our choices: Cheerios, Cocoa Crispi's, Kicks, Captain Crunch, Granola, Fruity Pebbles, Frosted Mini-Wheats, Raisin Bran, Grapenuts; all cereals with FHI of less than 1.0. But fear not, we can use our rulers to find our way through this over-sugared, artificially colored, chemically flavored, highly preserved jungle of American breakfast cereals.

Start with the product that has been advertised as the most wholesome Quaker oatmeal, small little flakes of smashed up goodness. These, like corn flakes and the like, are OK with an FHI of 2. But we can do better. How about bran cereals like Fiber One and All Bran? Small little cylinders of bran create the perfect breakfast cereal. These products meet the Skinny Food test with an FHI of 64.

Aha - here we find Ms. Smith in the cereal aisle - shopping for more Skinny Foods no doubt.

> **Ms. Smith - age 36** – *"You again? I know what you said about Cheerios and I agree. They do not score well on the Skinny Food diet. We do buy plenty of carrots and celery and other skinny foods, but my kids like Cheerios. So we will keep on buying them even though they aren't a skinny food. Some battles aren't worth fighting."*

Maybe - maybe not.

The next aisle over is the soda and chip aisle as well as the candy and nuts. This is largely a food desert for the Skinny Food crowd. However, even here, we can find some winners. Stick pretzels, for instance score a 100. We can also pick up a small bag of potato chips as our guilty pleasure food but as for all the nuts and soda, all are verboten. In addition to the chips, maybe we can find some leftover Christmas candy canes or licorice. And don't forget a chocolate bar, the thinner the better. Dark chocolate, 70% cocoa is a personal favorite.

Rounding the end-cap, I come to the aisle containing condiments, pickles, olives and canned vegetables. Nothing here to buy as they are all man-made and all in shapes that are quite unattractive. If you have an interest in pickled items, you can buy dill pickle spears or sauerkraut. Walk quickly past the mayonnaise, averting your eyes if need be. Can you really imagine eating something that comes in the shape of a quart jar? Yet, that is what the folks at the major food manufacturers want you to do – buy short, fat and thick in the middle, no thanks. The same is true with peanut butter and jelly - all in lovely chunky containers. While you are averting your eyes, take a quick peek at the salad dressing section. These are not fast foods, but fat foods. Although they come packaged in bottles that are taller that the mayo, they too are diet busters.

Ms. Smith seems to be following me around the store. Clearly, she is interested in how a Skinny Food "guru" approaches supermarket shopping.

> **Ms. Smith - age 36** – *"Look, you really need to stop following me, I am trying the best I can. You have already scolded me for buying Cheerios. But look in my cart. It is loaded with good nutritious foods. Sure there is mayonnaise, and guacamole dip, but there is also a chocolate bar and pretzels; good Skinny Foods. Sometimes it is hard to eat just Skinny Foods. We all need our guilty pleasures."*

I am not sure of Ms. Smiths's real commitment to the Skinny Food Diet. If we were to put her to the test and look in her basket, would we find donuts under the spaghetti? I wonder. When she goes around the corner I might have to take a look.

Moving along, I find myself in the aisle of pasta and rice, canned tomatoes and sauces. Here I can relax a bit, just a bit, as I find the ideal skinny food, spaghetti. Now for you noodle aficionados, there are many type of pasta: rigatoni, ziti, manicotti, raviolis, etc. But it is important to separate the wheat from the chaff and here we are looking for three fairly common types, spaghetti, vermicelli and linguine. There are many other thin types of pasta, and if you find a good Italian market, you will certainly have your pick of many long thin types.

If you do find yourself in such a place enjoy the experience of abundance. At Skinny Foods, we are all about celebrating life's little victories. Pasta, then, is our staple, the manna from heaven, brought down from above to help us navigate through the rest of this aisle. A bit dramatic you say, maybe, but hang on to your Angel Hair the worst is yet to come.

> *Police Officer, Scott Jones - age 42* – "Yes, I've heard about the Skinny Food Diet. I understand that there are many health benefits and it is a great way to lose weight. I really do, but you need to stay away from Ms. Smith and keep your distance from other shoppers in the store. You are not to go around looking in other peoples shopping carts. Got it?"

I got it all right, some people are just so overwhelmed by the inherent goodness of the Skinny Food Diet, that they can't deal with their good fortune. "Fear of Success," I think the psychologists call it.

Along with the pasta is often shelved the devil's spawn; rice, beans, dried peas, quinoa, risotto, cornmeal and the like. At Skinny Foods, we know that many other so called "diets" tout these carbohydrates as healthy, but look at what you are eating; poor, little, round or oblong seeds/grains. Is this what you want to look like - short and small, with sloping shoulders, and poor posture? We say "no" to those who would have you believe that these are the healthy choices. Don't be fooled, unless or until Hollywood plans on remaking the Wizard of Oz, I don't see many opportunities for Munchkins. So, don't become one. Stand tall in your thinness.

Exiting the pasta/rice/bean aisle as quickly as you can, head over to the meat department to see what is on special. Here among the "surf" we have some excellent choices. King crab legs, trout, salmon fillets, tilapia fillets, shrimp and herring are all good wholesome foods that follow the Skinny Food model. Stay away from oysters, clams, mussels, scallops and the like. Head over to the turf section for the strip steak, ham steak and flank steak, Skip the tri-tip, rump or rib roasts, fillet, New York and T-Bone steaks. Go instead for the spare ribs, bacon and link sausages. Watch out for the burger patties or otherwise as this abomination can be made into the number #1 enemy of the Skinny Food approach "Meat Loaf."

Working my way along the back wall we come to the dairy department. Milk and cheese are generally not on anyone's diet list. Loads of calories, loads of fat and milk sugars that the adult human gut wasn't designed to digest. In the "did-you-know" category, it is true that humans are the only animals that continue to drink milk beyond childhood, the only one. Why is this? We don't know, but at Skinny Foods, we are not going to embrace these easy calories.

After all, who wants to look like a cow or even worse a goat? No, we are going to be true to form and skip all of these dairy products. No milk-based yogurts, cottage cheese, sour cream, ricotta or crème fraise. However, if you are one of those folks who need to have cheese is your life and can find no alternatives; there is hope with one type of cheese. What kind of cheese you ask? Gouda, Cheddar, Jack? No, not these, but string cheese. Yes string cheese, long and thin and with an FHI of 128, it is an excellent addition the Skinny Food diet.

By the way, the police officer was a very decent fellow and we had a nice long talk on the way to the police station. He said he would try the Skinny Food Diet. Wow, another convert!

> *Judge Lenore Reynolds, age 61* – *"What can I do to get you to understand that your diet isn't for everyone? You need to back off and let them their own decisions. Even if the Skinny Food Diet is the best way to lose weight look and feel better, these people are adults and they can kill themselves if they want to. Since this is your first offense (California penal code 372 - Public Nuisance), I am going to give you 6 months probation and mandatory counseling. I don't want to see you back here again. Any questions?"*

Yeah, lots! However, I don't think Judge Reynolds was too interested in hearing any more about the amazing health benefits of the Skinny Food Diet. And clearly, she wasn't interested in improving her BHI score either. As a condition of my release, she required me to go to counseling sessions. I guess she wanted me to understand that other people have the "right" to be wrong.

> **Ms. Diane Payne, Ph.D., MD age 54** – *"OK, we've talked about the Skinny Food Diet for over an hour and I know how you feel about it. It is a great program and one that would benefit us all. However, don't you think that you are fixated on the Skinny Food Diet? You know, life is not just about diets and dieting. Next time, let's skip all the talk about Skinny Food and focus on your early childhood."*

In spite of the psychiatrists obvious concern about appropriate maternal relationships, she clearly recognized the value of the Skinny Food Diet. No doubt, after a few more counseling sessions with me, she will be recommending it to all her patients.

Chapter 7

TOOLS OF THE SKINNY FOOD DIET

We all love kitchen gadgets. Sifters, rolling pins, expensive French pots and pans, you name it, and I probably have it. At Skinny Foods, we like to cook. We are those folks who can whip up a gourmet meal without breaking a sweat. And whether you are a professional chef or just a beginner, you are in for a treat preparing your own Skinny Food meals.

First things first - start with a basic inventory of items in your kitchen. You should have an assortment of sharp knives, check. Pots, pans, cookies sheets, and baking dishes, check. Rolling pin, pastry cutter, measuring spoons and measuring cups, check, check, check and check. Mixing bowls, salad spinners, beaters, whisks, slotted spoons. All check. Of course, you might have a wide array of spices, flours, sugars, salts and oils. Put them on the back shelf for someone else to use.

In fact, many of the items found in your kitchen we won't use at all. For example, forget about using the casserole dish. It doesn't matter that it was a wedding gift from Aunt Bessie. Casseroles are not in the Skinny Food Diet, they just aren't. You might as well toss out the dish or offer it up at the next church bazaar. If you don't have what you need, you can always go online and purchase items from retailers like Amazon where you will find great selections that are reasonably priced.

To be a great Skinny Food chef requires patience and dedication. And just like any other profession, you will require specialized tools to produce some of the finest creations. The following is a partial list of specialized items that will make your Skinny Food experience more rewarding. Get them when you can.

Baguette Pans - We will be creating our own baguettes, pretzels, and bread-sticks. You will likely have all the necessary bowls, spoons, ovens and cookie sheets for the pretzels and breadsticks, but will need to buy your baguette pans. Check online for the best price.

Bathroom Scale - Here we are looking for the electronic style. One to record your weight in pounds or kilos or any other metric you choose. I like the ones that look like glass floating on the bathroom floor - very chic. Try and weight yourself every day at the same time, maybe first thing in the morning. Not only will you weigh less, but it will also motivate you to start your day with a healthful, Skinny Food Breakfast.

Calculator - You can use your cell phone (see below) to make the necessary calculations, but having an old fashion calculator isn't such a bad idea. One reason to go with the old style calculator is that you can make your measurement and calculations without having to worry about accidentally dialing someone's phone number when you slip the phone back in your pocket.

Cell Phone - However, you will need your cell phone to take a lot of selfies showing the world your new "you." Use all the social media at your disposal to announce your weight loss program. Give your friends hourly updates, letting them know the foods you are eating, how you feel about them and what your other friends think. And to incentivize your friends to join you on the diet, make sure you send pictures to the heaviest friend first. Include a cat video or two to keep the hourly updates interesting.

Computer with Photoshop Software- While the Skinny Food diet is truly a miracle, and guaranteed to help you lose weight, it may not be as quick as you would want. In this case, use Photoshop to make your picture ever so slightly thinner. BTW, this is not cheating, as these images are what you will look like in the not so distant future.

Gravity Boots - We considered the rack, but since there are few suppliers of these devices, we chose a device that can be purchased most anywhere. Check online retailers for the best deals. However, if you are handy around the house and like to build furniture, you might consider making your own rack. Check with ancient religious orders (if Wikipedia is correct, the Dominicans would be a good place to start) to see if they have plans or operating manuals you can purchase.

Pasta Maker - There is nothing like fresh pasta to make your Italian skinny food meals come to life. Making your own pasta allows you to create supper skinny fettuccini. You can go with a hand crank model or a fancy electric one. Whatever unit you buy, just make sure that you can set the pasta thickness for something that will allow light to shine through your noodles.

Photographs of Your Friends – Here, we are looking for candid shots of your friends gorging themselves on pie, cakes, donuts, burgers and beer. Any photo that shows their ample backside and eating unhealthy foods will do. Print out these pictures on 11" by 17" paper and tape them to the fridge. This will help keep you focused on the race ahead.

Skinny Food Diary - Here you want to create a journal of your dieting adventures. Day one will be filled with your hopes and dreams, what you will say to your ex-boyfriend/girl friend when they get a look at the new you and so on. Day five will be ecstasy at your significant weight loss. Day 10 will be heartbreak as you realize that you will have to buy all new clothes. Day 20, joy again as you meet up with the old boyfriend/girlfriend and their skanky pear shaped lover. Payback is so good!

Skinny Plates - You will want to get skinny plates to help reinforce you new Skinny Food Diet. No point in keeping round plates that will only remind you of your round self. Throw them out. Buy new plates, ones that are long and thin. Numerous studies have shown that folks who eat dinner from large plates eat more than those who use smaller plates.

Skinny Silverware - While you are changing your plates, you might as well change your silverware. Get skinny knives, forks and spoons. You will eat less and what you do eat will be more satisfying.

Straws - To make liquids score well on the FHI scale, we will need an assortment of straws. Go for the smallest diameters you can find and you will have the maximum health benefits.

Tape Measure - Here we want to measure our height and see how our height increasing efforts are progressing. Starting with gravity boots measure your height before and after a session. Don't be surprised if you are just a half-inch taller. With repeated sessions, you will gain the height you are looking for.

Wine Glasses - At Skinny Foods, we share in your struggles to gain height and lose weight. And, whether you are just getting started or a long-time SFD practitioner, we want to help you succeed. However you will need to be patient with yourself. You didn't to have a "Too Short" BHI overnight, and you won't be able to get to "Just Right" without any effort. Take a breath, grab a bottle of wine, your favorite straw and relax. Pinot Noir is a good choice.

Chapter 8

YOUR SKINNY FOOD DIET PLAN

As you can see, getting started on the diet is pretty simple. All you need do is buy some skinny foods, gather up a few tools, pick your target BHI, and begin. But, what should your **Just Right** target be and how best to get there? Great questions, and at Skinny Foods, we make it easy to achieve the results you want. Our 3-step process is your guide to creating the body of your dreams.

However, before you develop your Skinny Food Diet Plan, it might be instructive to look at a case study. We can learn a lot from others experiences.

A 35 year-old female, HK arrived at the Skinny Food Diet (SFD) office for a BHI consultation. Her therapist, who had heard of the SFD from the cousin of a former patient's mother in-law, referred her to our office. Good news does get around! HK was greeted by staff, weighed and measured 152 lbs, 5'4"; vital signs, BP 135/90, pulse 80, temperature 98.7, body type Endomorphic. Although she had extensive dieting experiences, there were four diets that we could be classified as significant (losing >25 pounds). Additionally, she had experimented with several prepackaged meal plans and hypnotherapy; in an effort achieve her desired weight. Based on an extensive interview, her diet history and current physical state, I classified HK as a "Yo-Yo type 2." While this condition was serious, she was not in imminent danger and I saw no reason to admit her to the SFD clinic. I believed that her case could be resolved as an outpatient.

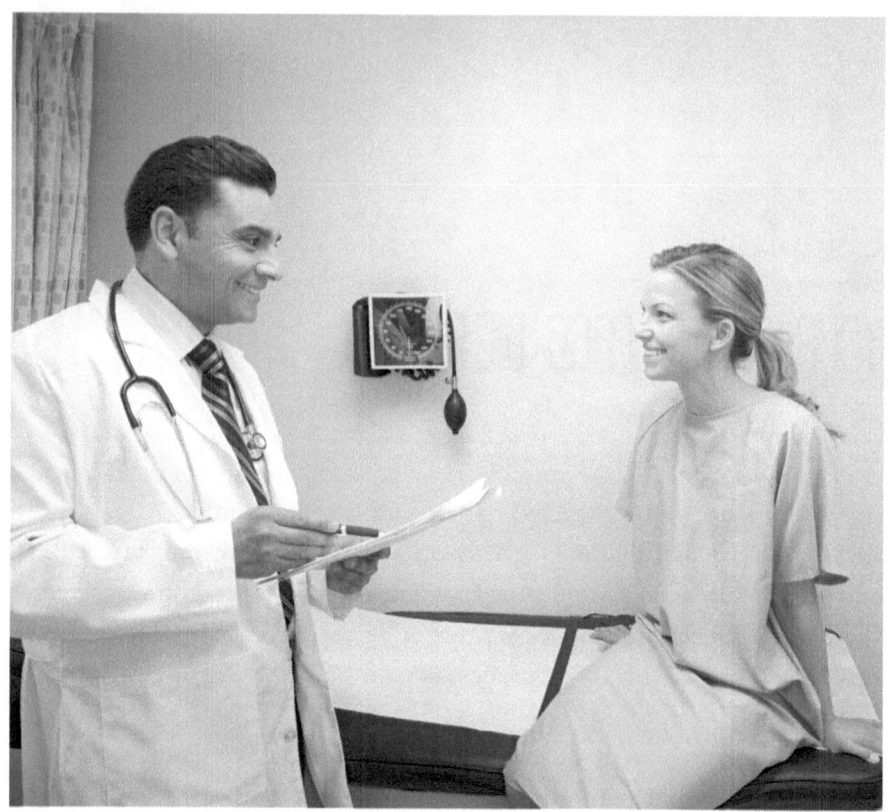

Visit to the Skinny Food Clinic

Referring to the BHI chart, HK needed to gain 3 inches in height and lose 22 lbs to achieve her desired BHI of 20.4 (height 5'7" weight 130 lbs). I prescribed an 8-week course of stretching therapy (12 hours per day 3x per week), 4 meals per day of skinny foods with FHI of no less than 10, and use of a straw 3/16-inch diameter by 8 inches long. I believed that this combination would be efficacious while allowing her to continue her daily routine. She was nervous about starting the diet, but upon further discussion understood the importance of the treatment and the need to begin immediately.

I arranged for a standard model rack (Hgt 34-009) including instruction manual and video to be brought to her house. On the days she was stretching, she was to use the rack in 6-8 hour sessions. I recommend that she use the rack at night while sleeping and/or watching TV. Timing is important because when your hands and feet are tied by rope, it makes it hard to cook, do dishes, laundry or other household chores. I advised her of a number of possible side effects including the potential for a significant change in her sex life.

For the balance of the stretching therapy time (4-6 hours daily) I recommend use of gravity boots. As HK worked in a professional office, I prescribed size 7 gravity boots in faux red alligator skin (very stylish). I forwarded a copy of HK's treatment plan to her supervisor and Human Resource director. I also ordered special office equipment for her, including inversion desk, anti-gravity mouse pad, screen and keyboard, and a gimbaled coffee cup holder. I advised HK's supervisor that "reasonable accommodation" was required to support her inversion therapy needs. Any questions should be referred to the local Equal Employment Opportunity Commission (EEOC).

Following 6 weeks of treatment, HK arrived at the office for a pre-arranged check up. When measure HK was found to have gained 2" in height and lost 14 pounds - an excellent result. She noted an increase in the frequency and intensity of sexual relations. Not surprisingly, HK reported her husband found the rack particularly titillating.

At the end of the 12-week treatment, HK was measured and found to be within a ¼ inch of her target height of 5'7." Additionally, she had achieved her target weight of 130 lbs. Both the rack and gravity boots were well tolerated. She did particularly well with the diet, commenting that the straw made it easy to consume liquids during both rack and gravity boot sessions - overall another successful outcome.

Wow, what could be easier? HK just followed the simple 3 step Skinny Food's process with amazing results. You can too, so let's begin.

Step 1: Find your current BHI
Step 2: Decide on your target BHI
Step 3: Choose the methods needed to achieve your desired results.

Current BHI

Nothing could be easier than finding you current BHI. Take a look at the BHI chart and locate the square where your height and weight values intersect. This is your current value and it will fall in one of three areas; **Just Right**, a **Little too Short** or **Way Too Short.** Note your current BHI score. This is your baseline and you might want to post this along with a cute animal video on Facebook. Let all your friends know that you will be starting the Skinny Food Diet soon and that jealously is not a pretty thing.

Target BHI

Here you need to get out some magazines and your sisters old Barbie doll to decide on your personal BHI goals. Unlike most political parties, at Skinny Foods, we celebrate our differences; so don't worry too much about your score. As long as you are in the **Just Right** zone you should be fine. For a point or reference, if the Barbie doll is scaled up to human size, she would be about 5'9" and 110 lbs. with a BHI of 16.3 - an excellent score.

Methods

Once your BHI goal is established, the next step is to decide on the best methods to achieve your increase in height and/or reduce your weight. To work on her height vector, HK used a combination of rack and gravity boots. This is a matter of personal preference, as either one is effective and are often used in combination. Like HK, you may choose to use one method at work and a different method at home. Also, if you spend a lot of time in meetings or at church, you might look for opportunities to get that extra bit of stretch, by installing a gravity boot station there. Many churches have found that once their congregants embrace gravity boots their weekly offerings rise significantly. Is this because of they are emulating St. Peter at the time of his death? Maybe, but more likely it is because being upside down is a convenient way to empty pockets.

The diet vector is just a question of eating foods that will give you the maximum weight loss. The higher FHI values of the foods you consume, the more rapid the weight loss. Unlike other diet book authors, I am not going to quote any specific values. You will not hear the words, "Lose 40 pounds in 10 days" from me, or any of the Skinny Food Diet staff. Not only is this level of weight loss highly unlikely, it can be dangerous. Research conducted with subjects *Lepus europaeus* and *testudo graeca* shows that slow and steady wins the dieting race. And so it is with the Skinny Food Diet.

To lose weight, simply eat foods that are in your Skinny Food loss zone. Once you reach your desired BHI, choose foods that will allow you to maintain target wieght.. Finally carry a straw with you at all times. You never know when you will need to "skinny up" a drink.

Now let's take a look at some of the best Skinny Foods.

Chapter 9

APPETIZERS

When thinking about Skinny Food recipes, we must start with the notion that they should be simple and delicious. No point in making things more complicated then they need to be. After all, the best things in life such as "revenge" are pretty straightforward. However, at Skinny Foods we are not "haters" and we take "forgiveness" just as seriously as "revenge." And a good thing too, as you will likely come across lots of folks who say that the Skinny Food Diet can't work or even those who question the underlying "Theory of Thin."

Instead of getting into a shouting match with these ill-informed folk, try to correct their thinking by saying something like, "If I agreed with you, we would both be wrong." Be as magnanimous as you can. It may take some time, but eventually they too may come to know the benefits of the Skinny Food Diet.

Let's get our "revenge/forgiveness foods" started with one of everyone's favorites.

Bacon-Jalapeño Poppers

FHI: 12.5
Servings: One - too good to share
Total Time: 40 minutes

Ingredients:
- 12 wooden toothpicks
- 4 oz (half of 8-oz package) string cheese

- 2 tablespoons chopped fresh chives or finely chopped green onions
- 6 fresh long skinny green chilies (4-5 inch minimum), halved lengthwise, seeded
- 4 slices of thin bacon

Preparation:

Heat oven to 375°F. Soak toothpicks in a small bowl of warm water to prevent burning. Grate string cheese and chives or onions. Spoon the mixture evenly into chili halves. Cut each bacon slice lengthwise into thirds (opportunity for extra thinness). Wrap 1 piece of bacon around each stuffed chili half; secure with a soaked toothpick. Place on cookie sheet. Bake for 25 minutes or until bacon is crispy and chilies are tender and the cheese is bubbling. Serve warm.

Grilled Garlic and Shrimp Skewers

FHI: 22
Servings: 4
Total Time: 25 minutes

Putting shrimp on a skewer adds an extra bit of skinniness to this recipe. This is a fantastic summertime treat. Marinate overnight for extra flavor.

Ingredients:
- ½ cup (8 Tbsp) unsalted butter
- 4 cloves of garlic, pressed or minced
- 1 Tbsp cajun spice (provides light heat; it's not too spicy)
- ½ tsp salt
- 1 Tbsp lemon juice (from ½ medium lemon)
- 3 lbs large or jumbo shrimp (12-24 count), peeled and deveined
- 12 medium wooden skewers

Preparation:

Soak long thin wooden skewers in water 30 min. Preheat grill to a temperature of 475'F. Combine all marinade ingredients in a small saucepan. Bring to a simmer then remove from heat. Pour one quarter of the mixture into a long skinny dish. Skewer 3-4 shrimp on each damp skewer. Lay skewers flat in the marinade. Brush with one half of the remaining sauce and refrigerate until ready to grill. (These can be made the night before, if desired). Place skewers on the grill and grill shrimp until just until cooked through (if using raw shrimp they will turn opaque when done). Brush on remaining sauce and serve.

Long Lean Wings

Food Health Index: 1.5
Servings: 6
Total Time: 60 minutes

Everybody's favorite football "game day" appetizers, wings of any kind are a Skinny Food staple.

Ingredients:
- **2** pounds chicken wings leave whole for extra thinness (24)
- **3** tablespoons honey
- **3** tablespoons ketchup
- ½ tablespoon red pepper sauce
- 2 tablespoon Worcestershire sauce
- 1 tablespoon paprika

Preparation:
Heat oven to 350ºF. Remove the skin from chicken wings. Mix honey, ketchup, pepper sauce and Worcestershire sauce in a resealable plastic bag. Add chicken. Seal bag and refrigerate 2 hours. Remove chicken from bag and place on a long baking pan. Bake uncovered about 30 minutes or until crisp and juice of chicken is no longer pink when centers of thickest pieces are cut. Sprinkle with paprika and serve with thin cut carrots and celery.

Skinny Salmon Bites

Food Health Index: 12.5
Servings: 36 pieces
Total Time: 20 minutes

Ingredients:

- 8 oz of smoked salmon
- 1 teaspoon olive oil mayonnaise
- Zest of one lemon
- ½ teaspoon wasabi powder
- 1 oz. pickled ginger
- 1large English cucumber, peeled and cut into long thin strips
- 36 small fresh dill sprigs

Preparation:

Cut salmon into pieces 4 inches by ¼ inch wide. Peel and then slice cucumber into long thin strips. Mix mayonnaise with wasabi powder and lime zest. Wash dill sprigs. Lay out on a flat space the salmon slice. Lay on top of the salmon a cucumber strip and then alongside lay the dill sprig and ginger. Roll the salmon tightly around the cucumber strip and place on a long skinny tray. Put a dollop of the mayonnaise mixture on top of the salmon. Refrigerate until ready to serve.

Extremely Thin Kale Chips

FHI: 160
Servings: One - you will want to eat them all
Prep Time: 30 minutes

Ingredients:

- 1 bunch (about 6 ounces) kale
- 1 tablespoon olive oil
- Himalayan Pink Sea salt to taste

Directions:
Preheat oven to 350°F. Rinse and dry the kale removing stems and tough center ribs. Cut into large pieces, toss with olive oil in a bowl then sprinkle with salt. Arrange leaves in a single layer on a large baking sheet. Bake for 15 minutes, or until crisp. Place baking sheet on a rack to cool.

Tapered Taquitos

Think about skinny pork, skinny cheese, skinny leeks and skinny tortillas. What could be skinnier and more delicious? Make these in advance for a Super Bowl party or even better, a funeral for you overweight friends.

Food Health Index: 8
Servings: 36 pieces
Total Time: 20 minutes

Ingredients:
- 1 medium leek, finely chopped
- 1 tablespoon canola oil
- 2 teaspoons ground cumin
- 1 teaspoon dried oregano
- 1 teaspoon chili powder
- ¼ teaspoon cayenne pepper
- 2 cups shredded cooked pork
- 1 cup (4 ounces) shredded string cheese
- ¼ cup minced fresh cilantro
- ¼ cup salsa verde
- 1 tablespoon lime juice
- 12 corn tortillas (6 inches), warmed

Directions:
In a large skillet, sauté leeks in oil until tender. Add the garlic, cumin, oregano, chili powder and cayenne; cook 1 minute longer. Add the pork, cheese, cilantro, salsa, and lime juice. Cook and stir until cheese is melted, about 5 minutes. Place 2 tablespoons filling over the lower third of each

tortilla. Roll up tightly into a tapered shape. Secure with toothpicks. Place taquitos on a greased baking sheet and bake at 400 degrees for 8 minutes - serve while warm.

Slender Spring Rolls

Food Health Index: ~2
Servings: 12 pieces
Total Time: 45 minutes

These refreshing rolls make perfect finger food for a spring or summer get-together; serve them with good-quality prepared chili.

Ingredients:
- ½ lb. shitake mushrooms
- 2 tsp. canola or peanut oil
- 1 garlic clove, pressed or minced
- 1 tsp. low-sodium soy sauce
- 7 oz. thin dried rice noodles
- 12 rice-paper wrappers, each 8 ½ inches in diameter
- 1 red bell pepper, seeded and thinly sliced
- 8 stalks of asparagus cooked till tender
- 2 carrots, peeled and cut into matchsticks
- 1 cup packed mixed fresh herb sprigs, such as mint, cilantro, and basil

Directions:
Clean and wash the mushrooms trimming off and discarding the caps. In a large nonstick fry pan over medium-high heat, warm 1 ½ tsp. of the oil. Add garlic and mushrooms and sauté for 3-4 minutes. Transfer to a bowl; set aside. Bring a pot of water to a boil over high heat. Add the noodles, stir and cook until tender, 3 to 5 minutes or according to the package instructions. Drain in a colander.

Fill a large, shallow bowl with very hot tap water. Soak the rice-paper wrappers, 1 or 2 at a time, until flexible, about 30 seconds. Shake off any excess water and stack the wrappers on a plate. Place 1 wrapper flat on a work surface. Arrange a combination of noodles, bell pepper, asparagus, mushrooms, carrots and herbs across the center of the wrapper; fold the ends in over the filling and then roll up tightly from the edge closest to you. Repeat to make the remaining rolls. Cut the rolls in half on the diagonal and serve immediately. Makes 12 rolls.

Chapter 10

FRUITS AND VEGETABLES

Nothing says "summer" like some freshly picked vegetables from the garden. Make sure to plant lots of Skinny vegetables. Skip the tomatoes, melons and broccoli. Do you want to really look like any of these? Focus on the green or yellow beans, long peppers, Chinese eggplant, and asparagus. Study these recipes over the long cold nights of winter and once summer arrives, you will be ready to go.

Grilled Summer Vegetables

Food Health Index: ~32
Servings: 6
Total Time: 20 minutes

Ingredients:
- 2 tbs olive oil
- 2 large thin zucchini, sliced
- 2 Chinese eggplant, halved and sliced
- 2 large leeks, sliced
- 1 long red pepper,
- 1 bulb garlic, cut into long thin pieces
- Sprigs of basil leaves, to garnish

Directions:

Place your grill pan on a gas or briquette barbeque to pre-heat. In a bowl, toss the vegetables and oil until covered. Grill the vegetables in batches until charred on both sides. Arrange the zucchini and eggplant out on plates. Top with the red pepper, leeks and the garlic cloves to one side. Garnish with basil sprigs before serving.

Spaghetti Squash

Food Health Index: ~160
Servings: 6
Total Time: 80 minutes

Ingredients:

- **1** medium spaghetti squash (2 to 3 pounds)

Preparation:

Preheat the oven to 425 degrees while you prep the squash. Use a large chef's knife and cut the spaghetti squash lengthwise. Spaghetti squash are tough so be careful with the knife. (Note: a trip to the emergency room adds extra time to this recipe). Use a small spoon to scrape out the seeds and bits of flesh from inside the squash. Discard the seeds (They are delicious but not on the diet. However if you must have a guilty pleasure you can coat them with olive oil and salt and roast on a cookie sheet for 10 minutes. Cool and store in an airtight container.)

Place the squash halves cut-side down in a roasting pan. Cook for 60 minutes or until tender and you can pull apart the flesh with a fork. Rake your fork in the same direction as the strands to make the longest "noodles." Serve the squash immediately, tossed with a little pesto or marinara sauce.

Stir-Fried Green Beans

Food Health Index: 119
Servings: 6
Total Time: 20 minutes

Ingredients:
- Himalayan Pink Sea Salt
- 2 pounds string beans, trimmed
- 4 tablespoons vegetable oil
- 4 medium-size garlic cloves, minced

Preparation:
Bring a large pot of salted water to a boil, and fill a large bowl with ice water. Working in two batches, boil beans until just tender, but still crisp and bright green. Start testing after 4 minutes or so, being careful not to overcook. When done, plunge beans into ice water to stop cooking.

When ready to serve, heat 2 tablespoons oil in a wok or large skillet over high heat. Add half the beans and half the garlic, and cook, stirring and tossing constantly, until beans are heated and garlic are softened and aromatic. Sprinkle with salt, and remove to a serving dish. Repeat with remaining oil, beans, and garlic. Serve.

Roasted Carrots and Parsnips

Food Health Index: 32
Servings: 6
Total Time: 50 minutes

This is so simple to make, yet so complex in flavor. Super-thin carrots drizzled in balsamic vinegar, then roasted in the oven and sprinkled with parsley and coarse salt. A family favorite!

Ingredients:
- 1.5 pounds whole baby carrots and parsnips
- 2 tablespoons olive oil

- 2 tablespoons balsamic vinegar
- Dash of coarse salt
- Dash of pepper
- Dried or fresh parsley

Directions:

Preheat oven to 400 degree F. Spray with non-stick cooking spray. Slice parsnips lengthwise or to matchstick size (to get an extra measure of thinness). Place on cookie sheet along with carrots and drizzle with olive oil and balsamic vinegar. Place in oven and roast for about 30 to 40 minutes or until tender. Remove from oven and place on skinny serving plate. Salt and pepper to taste.

Broiled Thin Asparagus

Food Health Index: 128
Servings: 6
Total Time: 20 minutes

Ingredients:

- ½ pounds thin asparagus spears, trimmed
- 2 tablespoons extra-virgin olive oil, divided
- ½ teaspoon kosher salt, divided
- Cooking spray
- 1 tablespoon red wine vinegar
- ½ teaspoon Dijon mustard
- ¼ teaspoon freshly ground black pepper
- 1 garlic clove, minced
- ¼ cup small basil leaves

Preparation:

Preheat broiler to low heat. Place asparagus in a shallow, but long, thin baking dish. Add 1 tablespoon of oil and ¼ teaspoon of salt, tossing well to coat. Place asparagus in oven under hot broiler elements for 4 minutes or until crisp-tender, turning after 2 minutes. Combine remaining salt, vinegar, and next 3 ingredients (through garlic); stir with a whisk. Slowly pour remaining 2 tablespoons oil into vinegar mixture, stirring constantly with a whisk. Arrange asparagus on a long thin serving platter; drizzle with the vinaigrette.

Quick Stir-Fried Snow Peas

Food Health Index: ~15
Servings: 6
Total Time: 15 minutes

Ingredients:

- 3 tablespoons peanut oil
- ½ pounds snow or sugar snap peas, washed and trimmed
- 1 teaspoon dark sesame oil
- 1 tablespoon minced ginger
- 1 tablespoon minced garlic
- 2 tablespoons soy sauce

Preparation:

Place 2 tablespoons of peanut oil in a large, deep skillet or wok and turn heat to high. When it begins to smoke, toss in peas and cook, stirring almost constantly, until they are glossy, bright green and begin to show a few brown spots, about 5 minutes. Meanwhile, in a small pot over low heat, warm remaining peanut oil with sesame oil.

When peas are almost done, stir in ginger and garlic, and cook another minute or so. Turn off heat and remove peas to a platter. Drizzle with heated oils and soy sauce. Taste and adjust seasoning, and serve.

Skinny Smoothie

Food Health Index: 120 (with straw)
Servings: 6
Total Time: 20 minutes

Kale is one of the world's healthiest foods because it is full of vitamins, fiber, and antioxidants. If you are on the go, use this smoothie to carry a dose of goodness with you. The sweetness of bananas and carrots will please even those picky eaters in your life.

Ingredients:
- 2 cups chopped kale
- 2 bananas, peeled and frozen
- 2 carrots, peeled and cut into sections
- 2 stalks celery, cut into sections
- 1 cup of unsweetened almond, coconut, or soy milk

Preparation:
Place the ingredients in a blender and mix until smooth. If necessary, you can start with the milk and bananas, then add the other ingredients one-by-one.

Caesar Salad

Food Health Index: ~60
Servings: 2
Total Time: 10 minutes

You too can make a great-tasting Caesar salad at home. This one has olive oil, lemon juice, anchovies, romaine and Parmesan cheese--everything you need to capture that classic taste.

Ingredients:
- ⅓ cup olive or vegetable oil
- 3 tablespoons lemon juice
- 1 can of anchovies fillets skin on
- 1tsp. anchovy paste
- 1 teaspoon Worcestershire sauce
- ¼ teaspoon ground mustard
- 2 garlic cloves, chopped
- 1 large head of romaine, torn into bite-size pieces
- 1 cup garlic-flavored breadstick croutons
- ⅓ cup grated Parmesan cheese
- Freshly ground pepper

Preparation:
Mix oil, lemon juice, anchovy paste, Worcestershire sauce, salt, mustard and garlic in salad bowl. Add romaine; toss until coated. Sprinkle with croutons, cheese and pepper; toss. As you serve the salad add a few anchovies fillets to each plate.

Plantains

Food Health Index: ~32
Servings: 2
Total Time: 10 minutes

Ingredients:
- 2 whole black plantains
- 1 cup Vegetable Oil
- Himalayan Pink Sea Salt

Preparation:
Pour oil in frying pan and turn burner on high. Slice plantains length-wise in ½-inch pieces (about 6 per plantain). Once oil is hot, place plantains in oil and fry one minute on each side or until golden brown with some hints of caramel color. Serve on platter with toppings of your choice.

Chapter 11

PASTAS

When it comes Skinny Foods there is nothing better than pasta. For those who grew up in Italy, you know the amazing variety of thin pasta, those with FHI >100. If you were lucky, you learned the art of thin pasta in nanna's kitchen. And because we love our grandmothers cooking so much we can even overlook their gnocchi's (FHI ~0.01). And because they loved us, they would have gotten the whole family on the *Dieta Margra* (Skinny Food Diet). No lasagna, ravioli or tortellini for this family. Instead, they would dine on heaping plates of spaghetti, vermicelli or an occasional manicotti or cannelloni. Sound good - *Andiamo a Mangiare!*

Spaghetti Alla Carbonara

FHI: 170
Servings: 4 to 6
Prep Time: 30 minutes

Ingredients:
- 1 pound spaghetti
- 8 ounces bacon, (long strips for extra thinness)
- 4 large eggs
- ½ cup freshly grated Romano Cheese
- ½ cup freshly grated Parmesan Cheese
- Freshly cracked black pepper
- ½ cup of chicken stock or bullion
- Himalayan Pink Sea salt

Preparation:

Bring about 8 quarts of water to a boil, add spaghetti and cook as directed on the package (8 to 10 minutes or slightly less if you prefer your pasta al dente). Pour the pasta and water into a colander and let drain. While the pasta is cooking, heat a large skillet over medium heat. Add the bacon and sauté until the meat is just crispy. Remove from skillet placing on paper towels to absorb the bacon fat. When cool, crumble the bacon into small pieces. In a small bowl beat the eggs and then adding the cheeses until well combined.

Return the pan to medium heat, and add the chicken stock and spaghetti. Once the stock has begun to boil, reduce the volume of liquid by half and then remove the pan from the heat. Rapidly add the egg mixture and stir quickly until the egg and cheese mixture thicken. Season freshly cracked black pepper. Serve immediately.

Spinach and String Cheese Stuffed Manicotti

FHI: ~12.5
Servings: 4 to 6
Prep Time: 30 minutes

Ingredients:

- 1 (10 ounce) package frozen spinach, thawed, squeezed and then patted dry
- 8 ounces shredded string cheese
- 15 ounces ricotta cheese
- 4 ounces cream cheese
- ½ cup shredded Romano or Parmesan cheese
- 2 eggs
- ½ teaspoon Himalayan Pink Sea salt
- ¼ teaspoon freshly ground black pepper
- 1 box (12 to 14 shells) manicotti noodles
- 3 to 4 cups marinara sauce (make it yourself from you favorite recipe or use 1 jar + a little more)
- ½ cup shredded Romano or Parmesan cheese, for topping

Preparation:

Preheat oven to 350 degrees F. In a large bowl, mix spinach, cheeses, eggs, salt, and pepper. Stir together until well blended. Place about 1 ½ cups of marinara sauce in a 9 x 13-inch pan. Spread it around to cover the bottom. Place the mixed filling into a large plastic bag (the ones that your news paper boy delivers your morning paper are perfect, long and thin). Squeeze the contents down to the bottom of the bag and then using s scissor to cut off one end making a ½ inch diameter hole. Hold an uncooked manicotti shell in your left hand, if you are right handed or in your right hand if you are a lefty and squeeze the filling inside the shell.

Place the filled shell into the sauce-lined pan. Repeat with remaining manicotti shells and arrange in the baking pan. Cover the pasta with remaining marinara sauce. Sprinkle ½ cup of Romano/Parmesan on top. Bake the pan covered with foil for 50 minutes. Remove foil and bake an additional 10 minutes until the cheese starts to brown.

"Long"uini with Squid

FHI: ~50
Servings: 4 to 6
Prep Time: 30 minutes

Ingredients:

- 8 oz. of linguini pasta
- 8 oz. of frozen squid
- 1 tablespoon of olive oil
- 1 leek chopped
- 2 garlic cloves, minced
- 1 (450 g) can of chopped tomatoes
- 1 lemon
- 1 handful of finely chopped parsley
- 1 eight oz bottle of clam juice
- Himalayan Pink Sea salt
- Freshly ground black pepper

Preparation:

Bring a big pot of water to a simmer, clean the squid and cook for 1 hour. When done, drain the water and gently wash them under warm water. Wash off any skin and remove the cartilage membrane. Heat olive oil in a heavy skillet. Add the leeks first and cook for 2-3 minutes then add the garlic and sauté until soft. Add the tomatoes, stir and simmer. Add the squid, and clam juice simmer on medium heat for about 20 to 30 minutes, until the sauce thickens. In a large pot, cook spaghetti as directed. When the spaghetti is done, pour into a colander to drain and then return to the pot. Add the squid sauce mixing until well covered. Transfer the spaghetti to a serving bowl squeezing with lemon juice. Serve immediately.

Shrimp Scampi

FHI: ~100
Servings: 4 to 6
Prep Time: 30 minutes

Ingredients:
- 1 pound dry capellini (angle hair) pasta
- 10 oz. peeled and deveined shrimp
- 3 tbsp. extra virgin olive oil
- 1 tbsp. butter
- 1 large mild red pepper
- 4 garlic cloves, finely chopped
- 2 tbsp. chopped leek
- 1 tbsp. fresh basil, chopped
- 1 oz. dry white wine
- Himalayan Pink Sea salt and black pepper to taste

Preparation:

In a large skillet heat the extra virgin olive oil and butter and sauté the garlic and chopped leek until lightly golden. Slice the pepper to julienne (see how we can take an ordinary round food (bad) and make it a skinny food all star (good) by modifying the shape) and add it into the skillet with the shrimp.

Sauté for 5 more minutes or until the shrimp is fully cooked (opaque and pink). Add white wine to the skillet and stir the basil and season to taste with salt and pepper. Boil the capellini according to package instructions, strain them and toss them immediately with the shrimps. Garnish with parsley. Serve immediately.

Scanty Canty "Ionni"

FHI: 12.5
Servings: 4 to 6
Prep Time: 30 minutes

Ingredients:

- 1 package of thin hot link sausage
- 2 tablespoons olive oil
- 1 medium leek, thinly sliced to match sticks
- 4 ounces mushrooms, finely sliced
- 1 cup chicken stock
- 12 ounces mozzarella cheese, shredded
- 2 egg yolks
- 6 tablespoons butter
- 6 tablespoons flour
- 3 cups milk (not skim)
- 12 Cannelloni pasta shells
- ½ cup mozzarella cheese, grated
- ¼ cup Parmesan cheese, shredded
- 1 teaspoon dried oregano

Preparation:

In a large skillet over medium heat add olive oil, leek, and mushroom cooking for 5 minutes or so until the mushrooms become tender. Slice sausage lengthwise to increase its thinness. Stir and cook all ingredients until the onion is softened and the sausage is starting to brown add chicken stock and reduce by half. Set aside. Then make a white sauce by gently melting butter in a medium saucepan. Add flour and stir until it forms a golden paste, the French call this a "roux". Slowly, add milk and whisk together until smooth. Continue whisking until sauce comes to a slow boil and starts to thicken add mozzarella to sauce mixture and continue stirring while slowly whisking in the egg yolks; mix to combine cover and set aside.

Fill a large pot with 3 quarts of water and bring to a boil. Cook pasta according to package directions (8-10 minutes), drain. Preheat oven to 400°F. Spread ¾ cup of the reserved white sauce on the bottom of a long oiled baking dish. Place sliced sausage leek and mushroom pieces in the pasta shells and then using a icing tube or plastic bag filled with the sauce (cut off one corner) fill the pasta with the sauce.

Place filled cannelloni in the baking dish and cover with remaining sauce. Top with shredded mozzarella and Parmesan cheese and a sprinkling of oregano. Bake in preheated oven for 45 minutes or until heated through; and cheese starts to turn golden. Remove from oven, let stand for 5 minutes before serving.

Pasta Pesto

FHI: ~60
Servings: 4 to 6
Prep Time: 30 minutes

Ingredients:
- 2 oz baby spinach - remove stems
- 3-4 Asparagus stalks
- Small bunch of basil - reserve a few for garnish
- 3 tbs. olive oil
- 2 oz pine nuts or sunflower seeds
- 8 oz. linguine pasta
- 2 oz. grated Parmesan cheese

Preparation:
Bring 3 quarts of water to a boil and cook the linguine following pack instructions till just tender. Remove the white portion of the asparagus stalks and then blanch the asparagus until tender. Remove from pot and put into food processor. Add spinach and basil to the pot of hot water After 1 minute remove the greens and then add to the food processer. Finally, add the olive oil and pine nuts, and process until smooth. Pour the sauce over the pasta and serve with extra Parmesan and scattered with basil leaves.

Chapter 12

MEATS

Protein is one the pillar of most diets and the Skinny Food Diet is no exception. We relish proteins in all its forms, and whether you are a vegan or carnivore, we have you covered. For those vegans who are overly sensitive, you might want to skip this chapter. We know that animal flesh is not for everybody and we embrace your choice. But before you go, recall the comedian A. Whitney Brown's line, *"I am not a vegetarian because I love animals; I am a vegetarian because I hate plants."* For those who enjoy chasing their protein, we have some great Skinny Food recipes for you. Let's start with everyone's favorite: Bacon Wrapped Hotdogs.

Bacon Wrapped Hotdogs

FHI: 3
Servings: 4 to 6
Total Time: 15 minutes

Ingredients:
- 6 hotdogs (longer the better)
- 6 hotdog buns (same for the buns)
- 12 toothpicks (2 for each hot dog)
- 6 strips of bacon (extra long)

Preparation:

Start your grill and adjust to a medium-low heat. Wrap each hotdog with one strip of bacon and secure with a toothpick at each end. One strip of bacon fits around a hot dog fits perfectly. Cook on the grill, rotating so that all sides cook evenly. When the bacon is lightly crisp, remove from the heat. Serve in hotdog bun with BBQ sauce, sauerkraut (the long stringy kind), or any thin condiments you like. Enjoy!

Hotdog Jambalaya

Speaking of hotdogs, a number of years ago, I was home watching a cooking show that featured foods of New Orleans and predictably one of the dishes was Jambalaya. As the show progressed, I thought that this Jambalaya looked pretty good and since it was just about dinnertime, I headed to the kitchen to get started on their recipe. I looked in the pantry and refrigerator for the ingredients I had seen on TV: shrimp, no, Andouille sausage no, celery no, and green pepper no. But I did have onion, tomatoes, and rice. I also found a package of hotdogs. I decided to substitute the hot dogs for the sausage and shrimp and finesse the rest.

As the Jambalaya simmered pathetically on the stove, I thought, "How bad can it be?" Well, as it turned out, it was pretty bad. At dinnertime, I scooped up a couple of bowls and handed one to my wife. Now, she is a supportive spouse and will generally try most of my experiments, however, one look on her face convinced me that it was terrible. After I tasted it, I said, "This is the worst Jambalaya I have ever eaten." If fact, it was so bad that we threw out the entire batch. It was a lesson in excessive substitutions to be sure.

However, "the Hotdog Jambalaya Episode" as it has come to be known, did serve a worthwhile purpose. Whenever my wife and I go to dinner and the food tastes pretty bad, we look at each other and mouth the words *"Is it worse than Hot Dog jambalaya?"* Thus far, nothing has come close and now we know what the "1" is on the rating scale of "1 through 10."

Fish and Chips

FHI: ~5 for the fish, 40 for the chips
Servings: 4 to 6
Prep Time: 30 minutes

Ingredients:

- 4 large potatoes
- 2 quarts vegetable oil
- 2 cups all-purpose flour
- 1 (12-oz) bottle cold beer (preferably ale or lager)
- 1 ½ lb boneless haddock or cod fillets cut into 2-inch-wide strips (5 to 6 inches long)
- Accompaniment: malt vinegar
- ¼ teaspoon of Himalayan Pink Sea salt

Preparation:

Peel potatoes and then cut lengthwise into thin matchsticks. This is the most important part of the recipe as the FHI is a function of how thin you can cut them. Deposit the cut potatoes into a bowl of ice water and chill 30 minutes. Heat the oil in a deep, 6-quart heavy pot to 350°F. Drain potatoes and dry thoroughly. Fry one-third of the potatoes at a time, stirring gently, until edges are just golden – about 4 minutes. Transfer with a slotted spoon to fresh paper towels to drain. Fry the remaining potatoes in 2 batches, returning oil to 350°F between batches and draining of excess oil. When complete, arrange in one layer in a shallow baking pan and keep them warm in the oven.

Measure 1 ½ cups of flour into a bowl, then gently add the beer mixing until just combined. Stir in ¼ teaspoon of salt. Dip fillets one at a time into the batter and then drop into the hot oil. Fry coated fish, turning over frequently, until deep golden and cooked through, 4 to 5 minutes. Transfer to a paper-towel-lined baking sheet and keep warm in the oven. Continue frying the remaining fish in batches of 4, returning oil to 375°F between batches. Season fish and chips with salt.

Chicken Satay with Peanut Sauce

FHI: 8 for chicken, 200 for skewers
Servings: 4 to 6
Prep Time: 30 minutes (total time up to 12 hours)

Ingredients:
Chicken Skewers
- ½ cup coconut milk
- 2 tablespoons fish sauce
- 2 tablespoons red curry paste
- 2 cloves garlic, minced or grated
- 2 pounds boneless, skinless chicken breasts
- 12 – 16 wooden skewers

Peanut Dipping Sauce
- ½ peanut butter
- 2 tablespoons honey
- ¼ cup lime juice
- 2 teaspoons chili garlic sauce
- 1 tablespoon soy sauce
- 1 long thin anchovy fillet
- 1 (½ by 1 inch) piece fresh garlic, grated

Preparation:
Chicken Skewers
Combine the coconut milk, fish sauce, red curry paste, and garlic in a mixing bowl. Pour into a large food storage bag. Cut the chicken into ¾-inch long strips (or longer if you want to add an extra measure of thinness to this dish). Add the chicken to the marinade and refrigerate for 2 hours. Soak the wooden skewers in water for 30 minutes so they don't burn. Thread the chicken onto the skewers and discard any remaining marinade. Cook the chicken skewers on a hot grill or under the broiler for 2 – 3 minutes per side, or until the chicken skewers are cooked through.

Dipping Sauce

Combine all ingredients in a small saucepan. Cook over medium heat stirring until fully mixed and warmed. 4 minutes. Serve the sauce with the satay.

Citrus-Marinated Steak Tacos

FHI: 4
Servings: 4 (2 tacos each)
Prep Time: 90 minutes

Ingredients:

- **4** cloves garlic, chopped
- **2** tablespoons fresh lime juice
- **1** tablespoon white vinegar
- **1** teaspoon crushed red pepper
- **1** small skirt or flank steak (about one pound)
- Canola oil, for the grill
- Kosher salt and black pepper
- Corn tortillas, warmed
- Shredded lettuce
- String cheese
- Green salsa

Preparation:

Combine garlic, lime juice, vinegar, and red pepper, into a large re-sealable plastic bag. Add the steak and refrigerate for at least 2-3 hours. Heat grill to medium-high. Remove steaks from the marinade and then grill the meat, turning once (6 to 8 minutes for medium-rare.) Let rest for 10 minutes before thinly slicing against the grain. Divide the steak among the tortillas and top with the lettuce, cheese, and salsa.

Lamb Chops

While tacos are good, there is nothing quite like fresh lamb cooked on the grill. Whether it is chops, leg, kabobs or even the whole carcass, there is hardly a more tender, juicy or flavorful meat. At the Skinny Food Ranch, we raised Dorper sheep and had quite a local following for our spring lamb. While it is not a good idea to get too attached to farm animals, we just couldn't help ourselves and ended up naming our first ram and ewe, Adam and Eve. After that, we named a few more including a ram with magnificent horns, Rambo, and then there were the twins Mint and Jelly. Another set of twins I remember were Rack-O and Leg-O, and finally we named one of our long time ewes, Momma.

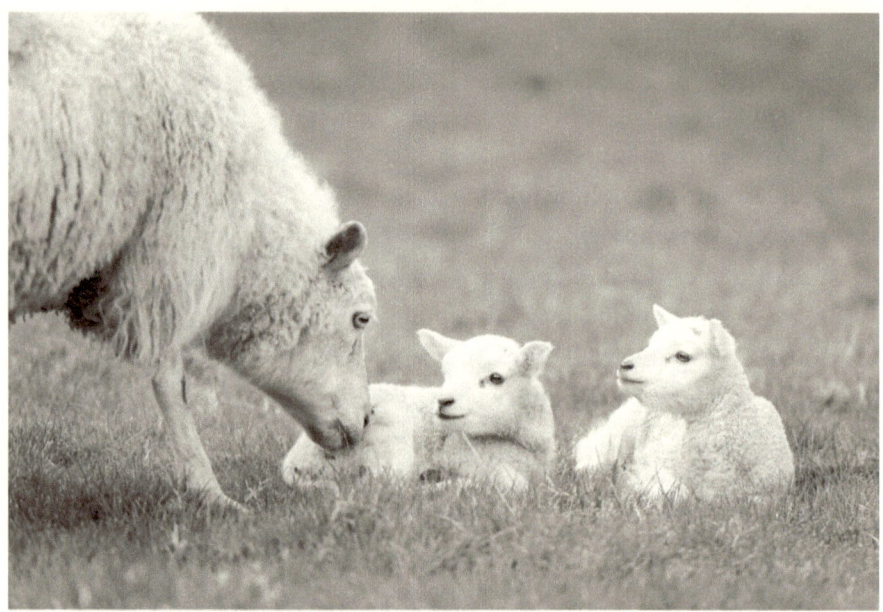

Momma with her lambs

Now Momma was not just a good mother, she was a great mother. And just to show how great she was, consider that she wouldn't give birth in the middle of a January rainstorm like most of the other ewes. No, she would wait until a nice sunny day in February. Well, all good things must end and after about 10 years on the ranch, Momma died. By now, I was pretty attached to her and wanted to find a nice place to bury her. As there was a magnificent oak tree down by our gate, I thought that would be the perfect place.

I loaded her up in the bucket of the tractor and headed down to the gate. After I dug a hole big enough to bury her, I paused and was thinking of how best to eulogize her. While I was contemplating just the right words, a car pulled up in our driveway. The car stopped and out comes a middle-aged, nicely dressed couple. At first, I thought they might be tourists looking for a nearby winery or directions to town, but they were Jehovah Witnesses who were in the neighborhood spreading the Good Word.

I said to them, "I am really happy to see you," which in their line of work probably doesn't happen very often. I relayed my dilemma about finding the right words for Momma.

The man was a little taken aback by my request and said, "We don't do that sort of thing."

"I apologize," was my reply, but really thought that this fellow missed a good opportunity to practice his eulogies, and he probably thought that I wasn't a particularly good candidate for the Jehovah Witnesses anyway. He gave me some of their pamphlets and drove off. As their taillights receded into the distance, I returned to the task at hand and again tried to find the right words to say about Momma. Should I recall her good years on the ranch, the number of healthy lambs she had, or how all the other ewes really admired her? There was much to choose from but somehow I thought that a simple service would be the best. And call it divine intervention or fate, but as I looked down at the pamphlet that the Jehovah Witnesses handed to me, I saw a picture of Jesus with a flock of sheep, so I placed it tenderly on Momma's side and covered her up.

Lamb Chops

FHI: 6-10 depending on the size chops
Servings: 4
Total Time: 1-2 hours

Ingredients:
- 1 teaspoons coarse Himalayan Pink Sea salt
- 1 tablespoons extra-virgin olive oil, divided
- 1 tablespoon white balsamic vinegar
- 3 large garlic cloves, grated
- 1 tablespoon fresh thyme leaves, lightly crushed
- 1 tablespoon fresh rosemary leaves, lightly crushed
- ½ teaspoon of coarse black pepper

- 12 lamb loin chops (1 inch-thick)
- 6 sprigs of fresh rosemary

Preparation;

Mix all ingredients except the lamb in large bowl. Add lamb; turn to coat. Place in a large plastic bag, place in the refrigerator and let marinate at least 1 hour (2 is better). Preheat a grill to high (or if going the traditional route until the charcoals are completely glowing red) and place chops on the rack, 3-4 inches above the gas burner or coals. Cook for 4-5 minutes each side till grill marks are seared into the meat. Move chops away from heat and continue cooking to desired doneness, about 10 minutes for medium-rare. Transfer lamb to a platter, add rosemary sprigs, cover and let rest 5 minutes.

Baby Back Ribs

FHI: 2-4 depending on the size of the ribs
Servings: 4 to 6
Total Time: 3-6 hours

Ingredients:
- 4 to 5 pounds of baby back ribs
- ¼ cup of Dijon mustard

Spice Rub;
- ¼ cup smoked paprika
- 5 teaspoons freshly ground black pepper
- 5 teaspoons dark brown sugar
- 1 tablespoon of Himalayan Pink Sea salt
- 2 teaspoons celery seed
- 1 teaspoon red pepper
- 2 teaspoons garlic powder
- 2 teaspoons dehydrated onion

Preparation:
Line a baking sheet with aluminum foil. Brush the ribs with mustard and then roll in the spice rub, patting the ribs to make sure that they are well

coated. Place the ribs in the baking dish and loosely cover with foil. Roast at 250' F for 3 hours. After 3 hours, remove foil and then cook for an additional 30 minutes. The ribs are done when the meat pulls away from the bone. Remove from the oven, and cover again with the foil, letting them rest for about 10 minutes. When ready to serve, cut between the bones to separate the individual ribs (long and thin, just the way we like them). Serve immediately.

Grilled Salmon, Braised Cabbage With Bacon and Leeks

FHI: 3 – 6 depending on the size of the fillet
Servings: 4 to 6
Prep Time: 30 minutes

Ingredients:
- 2 small leeks, sliced to long thin strips
- 8 slices of bacon
- 1 tablespoon of extra-virgin olive oil
- 4 salmon fillets (6 ounces each)
- Himalayan Pink Sea salt and freshly ground black pepper to taste
- 1 small green cabbage - shredded to long strips

Dressing
- 2 tablespoons of dark mustard
- 2 tablespoons of honey
- ½ tablespoon of fresh squeezed lemon juice
- 1 teaspoon of chopped parsley
- 1 tablespoon of white wine vinegar

Preparation:
Heat a large, deep skillet - fry bacon until crisp. Remove bacon and add leeks and cabbage stirring gently for five minutes. Remove vegetables and set aside. Add olive oil to the pan and when hot place the flesh side of salmon down and cook for approximately 4 minutes. Turn the fillets over and add shredded cabbage, bacon and leek mixture. Reduce heat to low, cover and cook for 12 minutes, stirring occasionally. Combine all the dressing ingredients

together in a bowl and blend until smooth. When the salmon is done, remove fish. To serve, place the vegetable mixture on the plate, drizzle with dressing and then place salmon fillet on top.

King Crab Legs

Even though you love all things crab, forget the body and go for the legs. They have the best meat and are a Skinny Food super star.

FHI: 20- 72 depending on size
Servings: 2-3
Prep Time: 30 minutes

Ingredients:
- 2 pounds king crab legs
- ½ cup of butter
- 5 whole garlic cloves minced and then crushed
- ¼ cup fresh squeezed lemon juice
- ⅛ cup of extra virgin olive oil
- Pinch Himalayan Pink Sea salt (optional and to taste)
- Pinch of dried parsley (optional)

Directions:
Preheat oven to 375 degrees. In a small saucepan, melt the butter. Add the garlic and cook slightly until it starts to brown. Add the lemon juice. Turn the heat to low and salt to taste. Add parsley. Remove dipping sauce from stove and pour into a serving bowl. Arrange crab legs in a long baking dish, brushing each leg with the olive oil. Bake for 20 minutes. Cool crab for 10 minutes and then crack and enjoy, dipping crabmeat into the sauce.

Iguana

In addition to traditional meats, why not try something a little different? One time, when my wife and I were traveling in Belize, we found a restaurant that served iguana. Now for those of you who have not traveled to Central America, iguana is a relatively common menu item. However, to make sure it appeals to the tourists as well as the locals, it often is advertised as "bamboo chicken." If you happen to go to your favorite Central American restaurant, and they have iguana on the menu, go ahead and order away. At over 4 ft. long, the bigger ones score a whopping 80 on the FHI index. Smaller ones are good as well with a FHI of about 20.

Chapter 13

BREADS

When it comes to breads, breadsticks, and their kin at Skinny Foods, we go the "Full Monty" leaving no bakery item unexamined in the quest for breadstuffs of a certain size and shape. Our quest is for gossamer thin crepes, angelic waffles, and breadsticks shaped like a garden hose. Granted there are some good attempts in your local grocery store, but to make them as thin as possible, you will likely need to make your own. And, at Skinny Food, we are here to help.

First up is the ever-popular Italian breadsticks, Grissini. According to legend, the baker of northern Italy, Lanzo Torinese, invented these bread-sticks in 1679. Clearly, these folks were early practitioners of the Skinny Food principles. The best Grissini are crisp and thin, and seasoned with cracked pepper, garlic, caraway or salt. You can even wrap them with prosciutto for a savory treat.

Rosemary Bread Sticks

FHI: 96 (+/-) depending on thinness
Servings: 6
Total time: I hour

Ingredients:
- ½ cup warm water (105')
- 1 package active dry yeast
- 1 teaspoon sugar

- 1 ½ cups all-purpose flour, divided
- ½ cup of whole wheat flour
- 2 tablespoons olive oil
- 1 teaspoon Himalayan Pink Sea salt
- 1 tablespoon dried rosemary

Directions:

In a large bowl, combine the water with the yeast, sugar and ½ cup of the all-purpose flour. Place in a warm location and let the yeast work until the mixture is frothy (about 15 minutes). Stir in the remaining all-purpose flour, wheat flour, olive oil, salt and rosemary and knead until smooth and elastic, about 5 minutes. Replace the dough in the bowl, cover with a kitchen towel and allow it to rise in a warm place for 1 hour.

Remove the dough from the bowl and divide it into four pieces. Roll out each piece into a rectangle, 6 by 12 inches. Cut the dough lengthwise into one-third-inch-wide strips and roll into even thinner cylinders, till they look like very thick yarn. Carefully place the strips about one-inch apart on a greased baking sheet. Repeat with the remaining dough. Allow the breadsticks to rise about 30 minutes until about ½ inch in diameter. Preheat oven to 400 degrees and then bake the breadsticks in batches about 10 minutes. Completely cool the breadsticks and store in a sealed bag.

As with breadsticks you can find some good pretzels in the store. However at Skinny Food's we found that most of these were too hard, too salty or just plain bad. No, we like home made pretzels. However to make authentic pretzels you will need to use an alkaline bath to poach the pretzel dough. Poaching gives the pretzels that smooth finish that makes them a favorite.

Pretzels

FHI: ~ 40 depending on size
Servings: 8
Total time: 40 minutes

Ingredients:

- ½ cup bread flour
- 1 teaspoon of instant yeast (no active dry or rapid-rise)

- 2teaspoons of packed light brown sugar
- ½ teaspoon of Himalayan Pink Sea salt
- 1 cup of warm water (105 degrees)
- Cooking spray or vegetable oil

Poaching Liquid
- 2 quarts water
- ½ cup of baking soda (see note above)
- ¼ cup of packed light brown sugar

Topping
- Large egg whisked with 1 tablespoon of water – for egg wash
- 1 tablespoon of coarse sea salt

Directions
Make the pretzels
In a large bowl, combine the water with the yeast, sugar and one-half cup of the all-purpose flour. Place in a warm location and let the yeast work until the mixture is frothy (about 15 minutes). Stir in the bread flour. Transfer the dough to a lightly floured surface and knead for 5 minutes or so until the dough is smooth.

Place the dough ball in a greased bowl and cover a towel. Let rise for 1 hour, until doubled in size. Remove the dough from the bowl and divide into quarters. Roll out each piece of dough until they are 6-8 inches long by ¼ inch thick. Using a knife cut into strips ¼ inch wide. As with the breadsticks, roll each dough strips with the palms of your hands to make them cylindrical and the diameter of thick yarn. Lay each strip on a cookie sheet spacing them about 1-inch apart, and let rise for 45 minutes.

Poach and bake
Preheat the oven to 375°F. While the oven in heating, bring the 12 cups water to a simmer in a large pot. Add the baking soda and brown sugar and stir until dissolved. Gently drop the dough pieces into the simmering water and poach for 15 seconds. Remove the pretzels with a slotted spoon and return to the baking sheets. Straighten any misshapen pretzels. Brush with the egg wash and sprinkle with sea salt. Bake for 30 to 35 minutes until the

pretzels are dark brown. Transfer the baked pretzels to a wire rack and let cool completely.

Baguettes

FHI: ~ 10
Servings: 12 (¼ baguette each)
Total time: 2 ½ hours

Ingredients:
- 3 cups of bread flour
- A teaspoon of Himalayan Pink Sea Salt
- ¼ teaspoon of yeast
- ½ cup of lukewarm water

Instructions:
Stir together all of the ingredients in a large bowl. Knead everything together for 3-5 minutes - the dough will be very sticky. Place the dough in a lightly greased bowl, cover, and let rest for 2 hours. Punch down the dough after the first hour and let rise again. Roughly divide the dough into three pieces. Roll flat to a rectangle of 6" by 12."' Fold width-wise two times to make a long log 12" by 2." Pick up the dough and gently pull it until it is about double in length. Fold the dough back on itself and then repeat the process several times pulling and stretching the dough till about 12" long by 1" in diameter. Do the same for the other pieces of dough.

Grease a baguette pan, and sprinkle the wells with course cornmeal. Place the dough in the pans and cover with a towel. Let rise for 1½ hours. Preheat the oven to 450°F. Just before baking, slash the tops of the baguettes diagonally several times, and spritz with water. Bake the baguettes for 25-30 minutes, spritzing the oven twice during the baking. The tops of the baguette should turn crusty brown. Remove the baguettes from the oven and place the baguettes on a wire rack to cool.

Yield: three 14" baguettes.

Homemade Thin-Crust Pizza

FHI: 1.6
Servings: 4 (two 10-inch pizzas)
Total Time: 1 hour 30 minutes

Ingredients:
For the dough:

- ¾ cups (6 ounces) lukewarm water
- One teaspoon active dry or instant yeast
- ¾ cups (6 ounces) lukewarm water
- 1 teaspoon active-dry or instant yeast
- 2 cups (10 ounces) unbleached all-purpose flour
- 1½ teaspoons of Himalayan Pink Sea salt

For the toppings:

- *For the base:* a thin brush of olive oil, pesto, or tomato sauce
- *For toppings:* you can use sautéed leeks, red peppers, mushrooms, dried tomatoes, cooked sausage, anchovies or bacon
- *For cheese:* use string cheese

Special equipment

- Pizza stone
- Pizza peel

Instructions:

Put the pizza stone in the oven and preheat to 500'F. In a large bowl, combine the water and yeast and stir to dissolve the yeast. Add the flour and salt to the bowl and mix into a shaggy dough. Turn the dough out onto a clean work surface and knead until dough is smooth and elastic about 5 minutes. Return the dough to the bowl and cover with a clean kitchen towel.

When ready to make the pizza, divide the dough in 2 and set one-half aside. Lay dough on parchment paper and roll it with a rolling pin till ⅛" to ¼." (At Skinny Foods, we only do thin crust pizza). If the dough starts to shrink back, pour yourself a glass of wine and let the dough rest for 5 minutes before you continue rolling. Roll out to a round shape approximately 14" in diameter. Repeat with the other half of dough.

To make the pizza, start by putting a few tablespoons of sauce into the center of the pizza and then spread it out to the edges. Add you favorite toppings, being careful not to pile on too many. (The pizza will cook much slower if you have been a little too generous with your toppings and the dough will likely burn before the toppings are cooked).

Using a peel slide your pizza (still on the parchment) onto the baking stone in the oven. Bake for about 5 minutes and then check the pizza and rotate if required. At this point, you can remove the parchment from under the pizza. Bake for another 3 to 5 minutes until the crust is golden-brown and the cheese is melted and starting to brown.

Remove the pizza from oven and let it cool. Repeat using the remaining toppings and bake the second pizza. To serve - slice into skinny portions.

This reminds me of the old story told by math teachers. There once was a young man who still hadn't mastered the concept of fractions and try as he might, he just didn't understand them. One day, when his mother was making pizza (using this excellent recipe) he said to her, "I am so hungry and that pizza smells so good, please cut it into 16 pieces so we can all have more."

Rosemary Flatbread

FHI: ~8
Servings: 6
Total Time: 40 minutes

Ingredients:
- 1 cup unbleached all-purpose flour
- 1tablespoon chopped rosemary plus 2 (6-inch) sprigs for garnish
- 1 teaspoon of baking powder
- ¾ teaspoon of Himalayan Pink Sea salt
- ¾ cup water
- ⅓ cup olive oil plus more for brushing
- Himalayan Pink Sea salt

Instructions:

Preheat oven to 450°F In a large bowl, stir together flour, chopped rosemary, baking powder, and salt. Add water and olive oil and stir until combined. Turn out dough on to a floured work surface and knead dough gently for 2 minutes. Divide dough into 3 pieces and roll out 1 piece on a sheet of parchment paper into a 10-inch round about ¼ inch thick. Lightly brush top with additional oil and garnish with rosemary leaves. Sprinkle with salt. Slide round (still on parchment) onto baking sheet and bake until golden with browning in spots for about 10 minutes. Remove from oven and place on a rack to cool. To serve: break into pieces and provide good quality olive oil for dipping.

Banana Waffles

FHI: 1.0
Servings: 4 to 6
Prep Time: 20 minutes

Waffles have been around for hundreds of years and are now eaten all over the world. We like to make them with bananas for a skinny breakfast.

- ¾ cups all-purpose flour
- ½ cup whole-wheat flour
- ½ cup sugar
- 1 teaspoon of baking powder
- ½ teaspoon baking soda
- ½ teaspoon ground cinnamon
- ½ teaspoon of nutmeg
- ¼ teaspoon of cloves
- ¼ teaspoon of Himalayan Pink Sea salt
- 2 large eggs
- 1 cup mashed banana (2 small bananas, overripe is best)
- ½ cup vegetable oil
- ½ cup sour cream
- 1 teaspoon of vanilla extract
- Vegetable oil spray

Preheat a waffle iron to medium-high.

In a large bowl, mix the dry ingredients. In a smaller bowl, whisk the eggs. Add banana, oil, sour cream, and vanilla and mix until blended. Fold the banana mixture into the flour mixture until just combined (lumps are okay).

Lightly spray the waffle iron with oil. Fill each section about three-quarters of the way full with batter. Close and cook until the waffles are golden brown, 4 to 6 minutes. Keep the waffles warm in the oven or covered with foil on a plate while you cook the remaining batter. Use your choice of toppings: butter, confectioners' sugar, sliced bananas.

Chapter 14

SNACKS

Snacks are one of the most overlooked, yet, most inportant part of any diet. Why, you might ask? Good question. The reason that snacks are so important is that they provide a Skinny cushion between your Skinny meals. Let's say, you had an excellent Skinny Food breakfast and you are looking forward to your skinny lunch, but for some reason, you are hungry mid-morning. No problem, just reach for your bag of Skinny snacks.

And, here comes the hard part, which one do you choose? Do you go with the jerky because you what something savory? Or do you go for the sweet and chewy licorice? Then again, you could eat some crackers or chocolate. Are those too many choices? Well, one strategy is to sample them all and see which one tastes good to you. Another approach is to ask your Facebook friends what they think. No matter which one you choose, you are in luck, because they are all Skinny Foods (FHI >20) you don't have to worry. Eat all you want.

Jerky

FHI: 160
Servings: 4 to 6
Total Time: Pretty much all day

Ingredients:
- 4 lbs London broil beef or 4 lbs flank steaks
- 2 teaspoons black pepper

- 2 teaspoons chili powder
- 2 teaspoons garlic powder
- 1 teaspoon cayenne pepper, more if you like it hot
- 2 teaspoons onion powder
- ¼ cup low sodium soy sauce
- ½ cup Worcestershire sauce

Preparation:

Trim all fat off meat. Cut steak across the grain in to 4 inch strips. The steak should be about ¼ inch thick. Note* if you freeze the meet and then partially thaw it is easier to cut it into strips. Pound meat lightly but not too much, (if you can see through it, it is probably too thin). Add all other ingredients in a large bowl. Mix well and add the meat. Cover and refrigerate overnight (8 hrs). Remove the meat from a bowl and place steak strips on baking tray. Set oven at lowest temperature. (150-175°F). Bake six hours, turning the jerky after three hours. Alternatively you can use a food dehydrator. Your jerky is done when meat is dried. Store up to 2 weeks is a plastic bag in the refrigerator.

Parmesan Cheese Crackers

FHI: ~25
Servings: One - too good to share
Total Time: 40 minutes

Ingredients:
- 2 cups whole wheat pastry flour
- 1 teaspoon Himalayan Pink Sea salt
- ⅔ cup warm water
- ⅓ cup olive oil (plus more for the pan)
- ¼ cup grated Parmesan Cheese

Instructions:

Heat the oven to 350 degrees. In a large bowl, add all the ingredients together and mix until you form shaggy dough. Remove dough from the bowl and place in large baking tray. Using a rolling pin, roll out the dough until in

96

fills the bottom of the tray (about ⅛ in thick). Using a knife, cut the dough in to squares about 2-inches on a side. Sprinkle with salt and bake for 15-18 minutes or until the tops are golden brown. Remove from the oven and let cool. Store in an airtight container for up to one week.

Licorice

FHI: ~140
Servings: 4 to 6
Total Time: 90 minutes

Ingredients:

- 4 tablespoons unsalted butter
- ½ cup granulated sugar
- ¼ cup dark corn syrup
- ¼ cup sweetened condensed milk
- 2 tablespoons (darker the better) molasses
- Pinch of kosher salt
- 6 tablespoons whole-wheat flour
- ½ teaspoon black or red food coloring
- 1 tablespoon anise extract

Preparation:

Line a small baking sheet with parchment paper and coat with cooking spray. Place a heavy 2-quart saucepan on the stove and add the butter, sugar, corn syrup, condensed milk, molasses, and salt. Turn the heat to medium and bring to a gentle boil. Stir the mixture frequently to reach a temperature of 240° F.

Remove pan from the stove and immediately stir in the flour and black/red food coloring. Once they're fully incorporated, stir in the anise extract. Pour the mixture into a baking sheet and let it set in the fridge for 30 minutes. Slice it into glorious long thin strips and twist into ropes.

Spicy Granola Bars

FHI: 3.4
Servings: 4 to 6
Total Time: 90 minutes

Oats are long skinny grains. In this recipe, they are combined with skinny nuts and seeds. The added spices make these granola bars taste like old-fashioned gingerbread cookies.

Ingredients:
- Butter, for greasing dish
- 1 cup of dates, pitted
- 1 ½ cup rolled oats
- ½ cup walnuts
- ¼ cup pumpkin seeds
- ¼ cup of Agave syrup
- 1 tablespoon of molasses
- ¼ cup almond butter
- 1 teaspoon of vanilla extract
- 1 teaspoon of ground ginger
- 1 teaspoon of ground cinnamon
- ⅛ teaspoon of ground nutmeg

Preparation:
Grease a 9-inch square baking dish with butter. Process the dates in a food processor until they have a dough-like consistency. In a large bowl, mix the dates with the oats, nuts, and seeds. In a small saucepan over low heat, mix the agave syrup, molasses, almond butter, vanilla, and spices. Heat, stirring constantly, until the ingredients are warm and well mixed. Pour over the dry ingredients and stir until combined. Press into the baking dish, and chill in the refrigerator for at least 20 minutes. Cut into skinny rectangles.

String Cheese

FHI: 128
Servings: 4 to 6
Total Time: 60 minutes

Ingredients:
- 1 teaspoon Himalayan Pink Sea salt
- One gallon of whole cow's milk
- ¼ rennet tablet or ¼ teaspoon liquid rennet
- Large bowl of cool water
- Large bowl of icy water

Supplies:
- A 6-quart pot
- Thermometer
- Colander
- Slotted spoon
- Long knife
- Small pot

Instructions Making Cheese

Pour milk into the pot and heat it to 90°F. Take the pot off the burner. Add the rennet and slowly stir it in for approximately 30 seconds. (If using a rennet tablet, first dissolve ¼ rennet tablet in ¼ cup water). Cover the pot and let it sit undisturbed for 5 minutes. A curd will form resembling soft custard. Using a long knife cut the curd in several directions creating 1-inch cubes. Cut diagonally as well as vertically.

Put the pot back on the stove and slowly heat it to 110°F, gently stirring to release the whey. Take the pot off the burner and stir slowly for 2 to 5 minutes. More stirring will make a firmer cheese. Pour off the floating whey. Pour the curds into a saucepan and then float the saucepan in the cool water. After 15 minutes remove from the cool water and float the saucepan in the bowl of ice water.

Once the curds are cool, you can begin making the cheese. First, heat a pot of water to 185°F. Ladle the curds into a colander, gently stirring and draining off the whey as you go. Dip the colander with the curds into the hot water for 20 seconds and then remove and stir with a slotted spoon, folding the cheese as you go. Repeat this process until the cheese become stretchy.

Remove the curd from the colander and stretch it like taffy. If it does not stretch easily, return it to the hot water bath. At this point you can add cheese salt, if you like. Continue to work it like taffy until the cheese is smooth and shiny. Pull cheese into long thin ropes for extra health benefits.

Chapter 15

SWEETS

We all love desert. There is nothing like long, sweet cannoli or crunchy biscotti to follow a great thin dinner. It is just the thing to keep you satisfied till your next Skinny Food meal. And what should we have for dessert? At Skinny Foods, we have lots of great choices for you. There is no need to eat the traditional desserts from your youth. Even if your grandmother's egg custard or fruit cocktail Jell-O was tasty, they are not going to make the FHI Skinny Food grade. I know this is hard for some, but this is no time for nostalgia.

And while we are at it, we should probably change the curriculum at the top pastry schools as well. It appears that pastry chefs are still making desserts shaped for the last century. It is as though they are living in the 1920's. Back then, the new new thing was a painter named Picasso. His "Cubism" style of art was very avant-garde, but a little hard for the average human to understand. Maybe it is just me but what is so attractive about cubes? They may be okay for ice or dice, but not for desserts. At Skinny Foods, we reject the notion that desserts need to be cubes. We are proud to call on the cylinder and the disk to be the shape of our desserts. Speaking of cylinders, here is a favorite.

Italian Cannoli

FHI: 12.5
Servings: 4 to 6
Total Time 60 minutes (plus overnight)

Ingredients:
For the filling
- 3 cups (22 ounces) fresh ricotta cheese
- ¾ cup powdered sugar
- ¾ teaspoon vanilla extract
- ¾ teaspoon finely orange zest
- ¼ teaspoon lemon juice

For the Shells
- 2 cups all-purpose flour, plus more for dusting
- 3 tablespoons granulated sugar
- ½ teaspoon coarse salt
- ¾ cup sweet wine, sherry or brandy
- 3 tablespoons vegetable oil
- Vegetable oil, for frying
- 1 large egg white, lightly beaten
- 2 tablespoons of powdered sugar for dusting

Directions:
In a mixing bowl, beat ricotta and powdered sugar until fluffy. Beat in vanilla, zest, and lemon juice. Cover with plastic wrap, and refrigerate. In a separate bowl combine flour, granulated sugar, and salt and mix thoroughly. Gradually add in the wine and salt.

Using your hands, knead dough on a lightly floured work surface until smooth and elastic, about 15 minutes. Return to the bowl and cover with plastic and let rest. After 30 minutes remove the dough from the bowl and divide into 4 pieces. Using a rolling pin, roll out the dough on a floured surface until about ⅛ in thick.

Cut into square pieces about 3.5 inches on a side. In a 4-quart saucepan, pour in 2 quarts of vegetable oil. Heat to 380 degrees. Wrap each round of dough around a 4-inch-long cannoli form, sealing with a dab of egg white. Fry 3-4 of them at a time until golden, about 1 minute. Using a wire skimmer, remove the cannoli from the oil to let drain and cool on paper towels. Repeat the rolling and frying process with the remaining dough. Spoon the filling into the shells and sprinkle with powdered sugar

Banana Crepes

FHI: ~4
Servings: 4 to 6
Total Time: 90 minutes

Ingredients

- 1 ¾ cups milk
- ¾ cup flour
- 1 egg white
- 2 tablespoons honey
- 1 (8 ounce) container yogurt
- 1 banana, diced
- ½ teaspoon vanilla extract
- Powdered sugar, optional
- Mint

Directions:

In a large bowl mix together milk, flour, egg, egg white and 1 tablespoon of honey. Place a 10-inch non-stick skillet over medium heat and spray with cooking spray. Pour ¼ cup of the batter into the skillet; swirling the mixture to evenly coat the bottom. After a minute the edges of the crepe will begin to brown and using a thin spatula loosen and turn the crepe over.

Cook an additional 20 seconds or until lightly browned; slide onto plate to cool. Repeat the process making crepes with remaining batter. As the finished crepes are piling up, use a piece of wax paper between them to prevent sticking.

In a blender, puree yogurt, vanilla and remaining honey in a blender or food processor until smooth. Remove the banana from the peel and cut lengthwise to make 4 long strips. To assemble, spread each crepe with about 2 ½ tablespoons of the yogurt mixture and add a strip of banana. Roll crepes into long tight cylinders. Place 2 crepes on each serving plate and garnish with mint sprigs and powdered sugar.

Chocolate and Mint Covered Pretzels

FHI: ~37
Servings: 4 to 6
Total Time: 90 minutes

Ingredients:
- 1 batch of large stick pretzels
- 1 12 oz. bag of Dark Chocolate Chips
- 6 candy canes, crushed

Directions:
In a microwavable container, heat chocolate chips at half power for 1 minute. Stir throughly. Continue to microwave and stir at 30-second intervals until completely melted. To make your fabulous snack, dip the end of the pretzel in melted chocolate and then place on parchment paper. Before the chocolate has a chance to cool, sprinkle pretzels with crushed candy canes and gently press the candy into the chocolate. Serve immediately or store in an airtight container.

Biscotti

FHI: ~4
Servings: 4 to 6
Total Time: 90 minutes

Ingredients:
- 2 cups all-purpose flour
- 1 cup sugar
- 1 teaspoon baking powder

- ⅛ teaspoon of Himalayan Pink Sea salt
- 3 large eggs
- 2 tablespoons Amaretto
- 1 teaspoon vanilla
- 1 teaspoon anise extract (optional)
- 1 cup whole almond, toasted and chopped a few times, not too fine.

Preparations:

Preheat oven to 275°F. Line 2 baking sheets with parchment. Mix the the eggs, amaretto vanilla and anise extracts in your mixer until well blended. Combine dry ingredients and then add to the egg mix. Remove dough from bowl and form into long fat loaf. Dough will be sticky. Bake until firm and dry, about 60 minutes. Remove from the oven and cool 10 minute. Use a long bread knife cut into ½-inch wide slices. Lay the slices on the baking sheet and bake another 30 minutes. Turn the slices over and bake 30 minutes more, or until the cookies are a light golden brown. Cool the biscotti on a rack and place in an air tight container. Store up to 1 week.

Chocolate Chip Cookies

FHI: 1.0
Servings: 4 to 6
Total Time: 45 minutes

Ingredients:
- 2 ½ cups all-purpose flour
- 1 teaspoon baking soda
- 2 sticks unsalted butter, room temperature
- 1 cup granulated sugar
- ¼ cup water
- ½ cup packed light-brown sugar
- 1 teaspoon salt
- 2 teaspoons pure vanilla extract
- 1 large egg
- 2 cups (about 12 ounces) semisweet and/or milk chocolate chips

Directions:

Preheat oven to 350 degrees. In a mixing bowl combine the butter with both sugars; beat on medium speed until light and fluffy. Reduce speed to low; add the salt, ¼ cup water, vanilla, and eggs. Beat until well mixed, about 1 minute. Add flour and baking soda; mix until just combined. Stir in the chocolate chips.

Drop tablespoon-size balls of dough about 2 inches apart on baking sheets. Bake until cookies are golden brown 12 to 15 minutes. Remove from oven, and let cool on baking sheet 1 to 2 minutes and then transfer to a wire rack. Store cookies in an airtight container at room temperature up to 1 week.

Homemade Thin Mint Cookies Recipe

FHI: 1.0
Servings: 4 to 6
Total Time: 45 minutes

Ingredients:
- 2 cups flour
- 1 ¼ cup butter, room temperature
- 1 cup powdered sugar
- 1 teaspoon vanilla extract
- ¾ teaspoon salt
- 1 pound bag of dark chocolate chips
- Peppermint extract to taste (about 1 teaspoon)

Directions:
For the Wafers:

In a large mixing bowl, cream the butter until it is light and fluffy. Add the powdered sugar and mix until completely incorporated. Stir in the vanilla extract, salt and flour until it forms shaggy dough. Divide the dough in half and refrigerate for 1 hour. Preheat oven to 350. Roll dough out pieces of dough until ⅛ inch thick. Using a cookie cutter cut out wafers and place on a baking sheet. Bake for 10 minutes.

Remove the cookies from the oven and allow them to cool on the sheet for a few minutes, then transfer to a wire rack. Repeat the process until all the cookies are finished. Place chocolate chips in a microwave safe bowl and microwave on high for 1 minute. Remove, stir and microwave on high for an additional minute. Repeat until chocolate is melted and smooth. Stir in the peppermint extract.

Line a baking sheet with wax paper, then dip one-half the cookie into the chocolate sauce. Place on the wax paper to cool. Repeat for the rest of the cookies. After cookies are completely cooled place in an airtight container. Store for up to one week.

Barquillos

FHI: ~50
Servings: 4 to 6
Total Time: 45 minutes

Ingredients:
- ½ cup butter
- ½ cup sugar
- 1 teaspoon of vanilla extract
- 2 egg whites
- ⅔ cup all-purpose flour

Preparation:
Preheat to 375°F. In a large bowl, mix butter with sugar and vanilla until light and fluffy. Gradually beat in egg whites, beating until well incorporated. Gradually fold in the flour. Drop the mixture by teaspoonfuls onto the baking sheet lined with parchment paper then spread thinly (thinner the better) with a spatula into a 3-inch circle.

Bake 15 minutes or until wafers are brown along edges. Remove each wafer in turn from the baking sheet, and roll around the handle of a wooden spoon until edges overlap. Gently remove from the spoon and cool a wire rack. Repeat with the other wafers. Store in an airtight container for up to 1 week

Chocolate Bar

FHI: 2.5
Servings: 1 (Why share?)
Total Time: Whatever it takes you to eat it.

For those of you who simply love chocolate and can't live without it, I have good news for you; chocolate bars in all their forms make an excellent Skinny Food snack. Heresy's Kisses on the other hand do not. Personally, I like dark chocolate with a cocoa content 70%. However, you are welcome to experiment to find the right combination of bitterness and sweetness. Maybe like me you will find that 50% too little and 90% too much.

Chapter 16

EATING OUT – EATING THIN

Although we enjoy making our own Skinny Foods, sometimes we just want to put our aprons down and enjoy a good meal out. We want someone else to do the cooking, the serving and the dishes. It is times like these that we seek out the *nouveau chic* restaurants, the ones with fun dishes and artistic presentations. While this type of dining is great, sometimes we are on the lookout for comfort food - a great meal at a great price. And then, we all have our favorite restaurants, places where we know the menu by heart, and where we are greeted by name. One of my favorite places is a local Mexican restaurant that serves a great caritas taco (FHI of 10). Every time I am in town, I stop in for a taco.

I feel the same way about lobster (FHI 8); I order it whenever I see it on the menu. But this raises an interesting question; in the quest for achieving the optimum skinny food result, can you overdo it? Can you consume too much of a skinny food, lose your taste for it, and then by extension lose your interest in life itself? To answer this question, I proposed the following experiment. My wife and I would travel to Nova Scotia, Canada, and for an entire week, eating all the lobster we want. I was of the opinion that you could not "overdose" on lobster, but my wife thought otherwise. To support her contention, she reminded me of the Aristotelian saying "nothing in excess". Maybe, but I liked Ben Franklin's version better; "do everything in moderation, including moderation."

With our respective quotations in hand, we headed off to Canada for a weeklong experiment. Now, for those who have not traveled to the maritime provinces of Canada, they are postcard beautiful. Peggy's Cove is a treasure, as is Lunenburg; but, no time for sightseeing, we were on a scientific mission. To accommodate our experiment, the good folks of Nova Scotia obliged us with lobster at every turn. Fast food giants like McDonalds and Subway even got in on the experiment with the McLobster sandwich and lobster rolls. Restaurants, bars, casinos and roadside stands all offered their versions of lobster as well. We gorged, dined, ate, snacked, nibbled, devoured and binged. Short of a feeding tube or an IV, we consumed lobster in every possible way. At the end of the week, I can say without fear of retraction that you cannot, I repeat cannot, over indulge on lobster. The last was a good as the first.

However, savvy readers will say that this experiment was flawed, meaning it was not conducted to the most rigorous standards, our observations were anecdotal and smack of "confirmation bias." Furthermore, to be of any true value to the academic literature of either the Skinny Food Diet (*macer cibum victu*) or the American lobster (*homarus americanus*), this study should have been done with a larger sample and "double blind." While we may agree in concept, it is hard to do a double-blind study where neither the cook nor the diner is aware of the food they are preparing or consuming. For example, you would be hard pressed to convince experimental subjects that the lobster they are eating is, in fact, a croissant. As for the sample size, I wholeheartedly agree, and recommend that readers perform the experiment themselves. In spite of the study's limitations, a draft of our research paper has been submitted to a widely respected journal and should be published any day.

Without digressing too much, what are the best items to order when eating out? Let's go back to our Skinny Food maxim, "If you want to be thin and sexy then eat thin and sexy foods." When looking at most restaurant menus, there are lots of choices, but often the choices are not so skinny.

When it comes to eating Skinny you must choose your restaurant carefully. It is unlikely that you will find a place that specializes in Skinny Foods. Oh sure, you might find some recognizable items on the menu, but a complete menu dedicated to Skinny Food, that would be extraordinary. We can only dream.

As far as other types of restaurant, your best bet is an Italian place with red and white- checkered tablecloths. If you can find one that offers breadsticks, then that would be better. Order all the linguini, spaghetti and manicotti you want. Order up a garden salad without the croutons. As long as you skip the lasagna, ravioli and macaroni you should be fine.

Other good choices are seafood restaurants; see if you can find one with a crab or lobster on their sign. This is always a good indication that thinness will be on their menu. Pick some skinny fish or you favorite crustacean, and order a side of French fries and coleslaw for a terrific skinny food meal. If you are interested in Mexican food, there are some good choices as well such as tacos and enchiladas that are not too bad. Definitely, skip the Nachos with a FHI of 0.5 because they not a Skinny Food. However chips and salsa are okay in moderation. Pizza is great choice as well. For extra FHI scores, go with the thin crust.

Nothing magic here, just choose your restaurants carefully, avoid the obviously bad foods, focus on salads and skinny vegetables, bring a straw for your 'before dinner' cocktail (margarita) and you will be fine.

Chapter 17

HOLDING THE LOSSES

For most of the year, we can stay true to the Skinny Food diet. We can enjoy our summertime barbecued ribs or hotdogs. We can cook up some corn on the cob, summer squash and kale chips - all terrific skinny foods. However, what do we do when the nights are a little longer, the temperature drops and skinny foods such as fresh green beans are harder to come by? It is then when our conviction to the Skinny Food principles are truly tested. And for the Skinny Food Diet, like most other diets, the supreme test is the holiday season.

When you think about holiday dinners in America or Europe what foods come to mind? Perhaps you like to enjoy a roasted turkey or possibly a baked ham. Just like image shown in the Norman Rockwell painting with the family gathered at the dinner table. A classic scene to be sure, but one that is full of calories, fat, salt, and round foods. Think about the poor turkey and ham, what are they really? Just overgrown meatballs with FHI of 0.50. Ditto for the mashed potatoes, dressing, cranberry sauce, grandma's rolls and fruitcake. All blobs of indistinguishable stuff and while it could be food, I am not really sure.

When it comes to holiday meals, we can make a little FHI progress with the pie and cookies. At least these foods have some shape to them, albeit round. However, it is only when we get to the green beans, do we find out way out of the holiday FHI quicksand and onto solid ground. No, holiday meals can be dangerous territory for Skinny Food Dieters.

It is not that Skinny Food Dieters are mirthless individuals, lack a sense of joy or don't share in the fun. It is just that we know what works and what doesn't. You won't find Skinny Food Dieters at the gym on January 2nd, trying to work off all the holiday excess. We won't be there, because we didn't gain all those "party" pounds.

To ward off the overly aggressive holiday host or hostess, I would like to share some Skinny Food Diet strategies that work well for me.

First: Bring A Straw

When you are handed a glass of champagne, eggnog or glögg and are asked to toast the New Year, use your straw to fight off the liquids corrupting influence. What could be easier? Straws solve so many problems; you might want to carry one with you at all times.

Second: When You Go Out With A Group, Specify A Designated "Diner"

This is the one person in your the group who will eat all the foods forced on you by your host or hostess. "More pate, with cheese curds on a stale cracker?" your host asks as they hand you this architecturally interesting, but unappetizing appetizer. Instead of begging off and pretending to have a toothache, simply smile and say, "Thank you." After the host or hostess moves on, hand this hors d'oervue to your designated diner. They will eat it for you.

Finally: Keep A Copy Of The Skinny Food Diet Book With You At All Times

Not only is it a handy reference, it just might be the inspiration you need in a time of uncertainty.

Chapter 18

SKINNY FAQ

How do I explain the Skinny Food Diet to my friends?
No need to explain. Eventually, your friends will have figured it out for themselves. They will scratch their heads when they see your smoother complexion, your new wardrobe, and the lightness in you step. They will observe you being kind to small children, strangers and dogs. They will likely say, "I wonder what is going on?" Maybe you have taken a secret lover, had plastic surgery, won the lottery or received an inheritance. No, No, No and not even close. Let them be jealous. You have made a positive change in your life by embracing the Skinny Food Diet. Even if they go through your trash, monitor your calls and ask the neighbors, they will not find the truth. The Skinny Food Diet will be our little secret.

Can I get too skinny?
No, as you can see from the BHI chart, there are no unhealthy height-to-weight ratios. As long as you are eating skinny foods, you will be fine. However, out and out starvation is not part of the Skinny Food Diet. No, at Skinny Foods we enjoy food and eat to become thin. It is that simple.

I really like using the rack, what happens if I get too tall?
This can be a problem for some. For readers who want to focus on increasing their height, the rack is a good method and sure to get results. However, if you stay under 8' you will probably be just fine. After all the NBA is loaded with tall players who make gobs of money. I am not suggesting that when

you hit the 7-foot mark that you try out for the NBA. However, that might be a good idea.

Should I do anything before I start the Skinny Food Diet?
Yes, before you begin the diet it's best to review your BHI objective. Other diets offer you the opportunity to lose a few inches, achieve better cardiovascular health, or simply be able to get into a smaller dress size. I guess these types of diets have their place. However, at Skinny Foods, we know the true purpose of most diets is to become thinner than our friends. Not so you say? Well, consider money, being rich isn't so much about having a million dollars, but rather having considerably more money than folks in your social circle. If you have a $1 million and you cavort with people who have $100 million, you are poor by comparison. It is the same for BHI. Being sexier than your friends is what dieting is all about. So, select several friends and let the competition begin.

Where can I go to find the skinny straws?
I suggest that you look on-line. I found a box of 10,000 neon colored straws for $10.49 (plus shipping and handling). These straws are ¼ inch in diameter by 5" long and that will give all of your drinks a FHI ranging from 29 to 80. (Mesomorphic body types score a 40 FHI). Assuming that you have 5 non-water drinks per day the 10,000-straw package should last you approximately 5 and ½ years.

Are snake and iguana available in my local store?
You might have to look for these items at specialty retailers, however it is unlikely that you will find them in most stores. As with many items, the Internet is your ticket to finding the best sources.

How do I determine if something thin is edible?
Good question. Here, American author, *Ambrose Bierce* said it best. He defined edible as "Good to eat, and wholesome to digest, as a worm to a toad, a toad to a snake, a snake to a pig, a pig to a man, and a man to a worm." Note his reference to the worm and snake, both excellent Skinny Foods.

I really don't like to cook - can I still be on the Skinny Food Diet?
You bet.

Where can I find a Skinny Food support group?
Go on-line to find your local chapter of Skinny Food Anonymous. Meetings are generally held on Thursday afternoons at 4:00.

I like some of the foods but not others - do I have to eat all Skinny Foods?
No. One of the most attractive features of the Skinny Food Diet is that you can create your own menu from a range of skinny foods. Think back to your high school math, specifically "averages." Say you really love meatballs, can't live without them. Then if you can put the meatballs (FHI 0.33) on a plate of spaghetti (FHI 200) the average FHI is 100.165, a great skinny meal. What could be simpler?

What happens if I cheat and eat a jelly-filled donut?
If you find yourself thinking about eating a donut or muffin, just recall that the Samaritan word for "donut" is "Gomorrah." And, we all know what happened there. No, if you find yourself weakening or questioning your commitment to the Skinny Food Diet plan, take heart. At Skinny Food we've got your back. You can:

1. Go off the diet for 2 months, gain a ton of weight and then spend 6 months in counseling to rediscover your inner thinness.
2. Attend a Skinny Food Diet support group meeting.
3. Take a picture of your left thigh and post it on-line to help you remember why you are dieting in the first place. Make sure all your friends "like" and/or comment on your picture.

Selected Bibliography and Disclaimer

In writing the title for the Skinny Food Diet book, I reviewed a number of other successful 'diet' book titles. As they are all guaranteed to help you lose weight and feel better, it is hard to know which ones are best. I have my personal favorites, (I particularly like the ones with rhyming titles). However, I leave it to the reader to choose the titles they find most attractive. Not so much to consider the substance of the diet, but the author's ability to convey the entirety of the diet in a clever turn of phrase.

While the referenced books played a large part in the creation of the Skinny Food Diet's title, the contents of these books did not. Any correlation of the Skinny Food Diet to other diets or diet books whether real or imagined would be amazing and purely coincidental.

The Stash Plan: Your 21-Day Guide to Shed Weight, Feel Great, and Take Charge of Your Health by Laura Prepon, Elizabeth Troy

Trim Healthy Mama Cookbook: Eat Up and Slim Down with More Than 350 Healthy Recipes by Pearl Barrett, Serene Allison

10-Day Green Smoothie Cleanse: Lose Up to 15 Pounds in 10 Days! by JJ Smith

Grain Brain: The Surprising Truth about Wheat, Carbs, and Sugar—Your Brain's Silent Killers by David Perlmutter

The Blood Sugar Solution 10-Day Detox Diet: Activate Your Body's Natural Ability to Burn Fat and Lose Weight Fast by Mark Hyman MD

The End of Dieting: How to Live for Life by Joel Fuhrman

The Doctor's Diet: Dr. Travis Stork's STAT Program to Help You Lose Weight & Restore Your Health by Travis Stork

Super Shred: The Big Results Diet: 4 Weeks, 20 Pounds, Lose It Faster! by Ian K. Smith

The Pound a Day Diet: Lose Up to 5 Pounds in 5 Days by Eating the Foods You Love by Rocco DiSpirito

The Hungry Girl Diet: Big Portions. Big Results. Drop 10 Pounds in 4 Weeks by Lisa Lillien

The Pound a Day Diet: Lose Up to 5 Pounds in 5 Days by Eating the Foods You Love by Rocco DiSpirito

Skinny Meals: Everything You Need To Lose Weight--Fast! By Bob Harper

Now Eat This! 100 Quick Calorie Cuts at Home / On-the-Go by Rocco DiSpirito

The Belly Fat Cure Quick Meals: Lose 4 to 9 lbs. a Week with On-the-Go Carb Swaps by Jorge Cruise

Dr. Atkins' New Diet Revolution By Robert C., M.D. Atkins M.D.

The Paleo Diet: Lose Weight and Get Healthy by Eating the Foods You Were Designed to Eat by Loren Cordain

Wheat Belly: Lose the Wheat, Lose the Weight, and Find Your Path Back to Health by William Davis

The Skinny Rules: The Simple, Nonnegotiable Principles for Getting to Thin by Bob Harper, Greg Critser

The DASH Diet Action Plan: Proven to Lower Blood Pressure and Cholesterol Without Medication by Marla Heller

Super Immunity: The Essential Nutrition Guide for Boosting Your Body's Defenses to Live Longer, Stronger, and Disease Free by Joel Fuhrman

Green Eggs and Ham by Dr. Seuss

Notes:

About The Author

An engineer by training, and a renaissance man by disposition, Caduceus Twigg always had the uncanny knack of being able to put two-and-two together. Using this ability, he pursued undergraduate and advanced degrees in engineering and business. He began his career at Pratt and Whitney Aircraft, where rocket scientists really do exist. He later moved on to help found a wind, energy start-up, then to an optics company, a silicon valley electronics manufacturer and finally to a community college where he is Professor of Business. In addition to his teaching, he is an accomplished foodie, chef, grape grower (Morning Wood Vineyards), olive curer, and sheep rancher. In his spare time, he served on the board of a local community health center and searches antique dealers and second-hand shops everywhere for the lost Picasso that we all know is out there, somewhere.

www.ingramcontent.com/pod-product-compliance
Lightning Source LLC
Chambersburg PA
CBHW020535290526
45786CB00002B/884